Comprehension of Wh-Dependencies in Broca's Aphasia

Comprehension of Wh-Dependencies in Broca's Aphasia

By

Vanja Kljajevic

CAMBRIDGE
SCHOLARS
PUBLISHING

Comprehension of Wh-Dependencies in Broca's Aphasia,
by Vanja Kljajevic

This book first published 2012

Cambridge Scholars Publishing

12 Back Chapman Street, Newcastle upon Tyne, NE6 2XX, UK

British Library Cataloguing in Publication Data
A catalogue record for this book is available from the British Library

ISBN (10): 1-4438-3666-4, ISBN (13): 978-1-4438-3666-1

To the memory of my father,
Radoje Kljajević

TABLE OF CONTENTS

LIST OF TABLES

ACKNOWLEDGMENTS

This book is a re-written version of the 2005 doctoral dissertation I produced at the Institute of Cognitive Science, Carleton University, Ottawa. This new version has been updated to include a more developed morphological account of the data that was only sketched in the original version as well as a number of research findings that have been published since completion of the original. The result, I hope, is a clearer picture of the comprehension of *wh*-dependencies in Croatian aphasic speakers.

The research reported in this book was conducted under the guidance of Marie-Odile Junker and Kumiko Murasugi, whom I would like to thank for their helpful advice and encouragement. I would also like to thank Jack Kelly, Monique Sénéchal and Eta Schneiderman for their comments on the reported research. I am grateful to Vida Demarin, Višnja Akrap-Kotevski, Zvjezdana Trifunović, and Marija Paškvalin from Zagreb for their assistance in finding aphasic patients for the study. Thanks are due to Don Ross for his editorial help. Finally, I would like to thank my family and friends for their encouragement during the preparation of this book.

LIST OF ABBREVIATIONS

Acc	Accusative
BA	Brodmann area
BDAE	Boston Diagnostic Aphasia Examination
CT	computed tomography
DAH	Direct Association Theory
DQ	direct questions
ECA	external carotid artery
ERP	Event Related Brain Potentials
EQ	embedded questions
EQ1PP	embedded questions with 1 prepositional phrase (PP)
EQ2PPs	embedded questions with 2 prepositional phrases (PPs)
f.	feminine
fMRI	functional Magnetic Resonance Imaging
GB	Government and Binding Theory
GG	Generative Grammar
ICA	internal carotid artery
lpt.	l-participle
LAN	left anterior negativity
LD	long-distance questions
LD *za*	long-distance questions with the preposition *za*
LTM	long-term memory
m.	masculine
MCA	middle cerebral artery
n.	neuter
Nom	Nominative
NP	noun phrase
OAA	overarching agrammatism
p.	plural
Pass.	passive
past	past tense
PCA	posterior cerebral artery
PET	positron emission tomography
PQ	passivized questions
pres.	present tense
RC	relative clauses

RCPM	Raven's Colored Progressive Matrices
RTDH	Revised Trace Deletion Hypothesis
s.	singular
SPLT	Syntactic Prediction Locality Theory
SOV	Subject-Object-Verb word order
SVO	Subject-Verb-Object word order
SWM	syntactic working memory
TBA	Trace Based Account
TDH	Trace Deletion Hypothesis
VP	verb phrase
WM	working memory

CHAPTER ONE

INTRODUCTION

1. Language Comprehension Architecture

Language is embedded in cognition and as such it is neither a unified nor isolated phenomenon. Many neurobiological and computational processes are involved in language processing. For example, speech perception and reading require perceptual transformations in the auditory and visual cortices (Hickok & Poeppel, 2004). Speaking requires motor control processes supported by the motor cortical areas, basal ganglia and cerebellum (Kutas, Federmeier, Coulson, King & Münte, 2000). Auditory language comprehension, which is the focus of this book, is carried out by several language subsystems, such as the phonological, semantic and syntactic subsystems, and is supported by memory and attentional processes.

The phonological subsystem of auditory comprehension carries out phonetic and phonological processes. Neuroimaging evidence suggests that this subsystem involves certain temporal areas bilaterally as well as the left dorsal portion of the Brodmann area (BA) 44 (Price, 2010). The semantic subsystem in auditory comprehension activates several areas, depending on the nature of the semantic task: while passive listening activates temporal region BA 22/42 bilaterally, other semantic tasks activate anterior and posterior parts of the left middle temporal gyrus (BA 21), bilateral anterior temporal poles (BA 38), left angular gyrus (BA 39), as well as left pars orbitalis (BA 47), pars triangularis (BA 45), middle frontal gyrus (BA 46), and pars opercularis (BA 44) (Friederici, 1998; Price, 2010). The syntactic subsystem involved in sentence comprehension activates Broca's area (BAs 44, 45), BA 39, the supramarginal gyrus (BA 40), and the superior temporal gyrus (BA 22) of the dominant hemisphere (Stromswold, Caplan, Alpert & Rauch, 1996; Grodzinsky, 2000b; Caplan, Vijayan, Kuperberg, West, Waters, Greve & Dale, 2001; Fiebach, Schlesewsky, Lohmann, von Cramon & Friederici, 2004). Computationally more demanding tasks affect the brain responses, resulting in variability in activation (Just, Carpenter, Keller, Eddy & Thulborn, 1996).

The auditory language comprehension also depends on the functional connectivity between brain areas and so the white matter pathways, such as the inferior occipito-frontal fasciculus, the arcuate fasciculus, and the middle and inferior longitudinal fasciculi are highly relevant for comprehension processes (Turken & Dronkers, 2011). Furthermore, there are indications that some subcortical structures related to rule-based elements of processing, such as the basal ganglia, are also involved in syntactic comprehension (Caplan, 2002).

As a higher cognitive function, language is supported by other cognitive systems, such as memory and attention. This further means that the parietal lobe, which is implicated in attentional processes, and the hippocampal, medial temporal, and frontal lobe structures, as implicated in memory processes, also support language processing (Kutas et al., 2000). Thus, many areas of the brain are involved in language processing and the relationship between the processing components and cortical regions is rather complex. In computational terms, it means that the processing of language requires resources from more than one cognitive domain.

Until recently, the role of memory and attention in comprehension and other language processes had been overlooked. Two steps were necessary to overcome this problem: first, it was essential to recognize that each of these cognitive domains makes their respective resources available to information processing, and second, it was necessary to define the nature of systems such as working memory (WM) that link cognitive information from different domains (Van der Zee & Nikanne, 2000). Indeed, growing interest in the role of WM in language comprehension has already created a dynamic field which incorporates theoretical knowledge, methodology and empirical findings from several disciplines (Caplan et al., 2001; Embick, Marantz, Miyashita, O'Neil & Sakai, 2000; Felser, Clahsen, Münte, 2003; Just et al, 1996; Kang, Constable, Gore & Avrutin, 1999; Keller, Carpenter & Just, 2001; Kotz & Friederici, 2003; Münte & Heinze, 1994; Stowe, Withaar, Wijers, Broere & Paans, 2002; Swaab, Brown & Hagoort, 1997; Vos, Gunter, Schriefers & Friederici, 2001; among others). While there is general agreement that without WM it would not be possible to temporarily store intermediate representations on which subsequent processes operate (which is crucial in any kind of syntax), research on the impact of WM on the comprehension of syntax of language (syntactic comprehension) has resulted in conflicting conclusions (Just & Carpenter, 1992; Martin & Romani, 1994; Miyake, Carpenter & Just, 1994, 1995; Caplan & Waters, 1999, 2002; Crosson et al., 1999; Vos et al., 2001). This is not a trivial matter, since it leaves open issues of theoretical framework, interpretation of empirical findings and choice of appropriate research methods. This is particularly evident in research on Broca's aphasia, a language disorder caused by focal brain damage, which is also characterized by limited processing resources and slowed access to linguistic information (Kolk & Heeschen, 1990; Prather, Shapiro, Zurif & Swinney, 1991; Kolk, 1995; Zurif et al., 1993; Frazier & McNamara, 1995; Swinney, Zurif, Prather & Love, 1996; Swaab et al., 1997).

2. Sentence Comprehension in Broca's Aphasia

Due to the effortful, halting speech Broca's aphasics produce, and their omission of function words (also known as closed-class words) such as auxiliaries and copulas, Broca's aphasia was originally qualified as a disorder limited to speech production. However, Caramazza and Zurif (1976) found that English speaking Broca's aphasics also had difficulty with syntactic comprehension, in particular when sentence meaning was not facilitated by semantic or pragmatic cues indicating thematic roles and depended on syntactic information, as in semantically reversible object relative center-embedded sentences in (1).

(1) The boy that the girl is kissing is happy.

Subsequent work has confirmed the finding, and in further examining whether the syntactic comprehension deficit in Broca's aphasic patients is manifested in other syntactic structures as well, researchers came to the conclusion that there exists a comprehension pattern of sparing and deficit in this population. The pattern can be described in the following way: Broca's aphasics show deficient syntactic comprehension in structures that include extraction from the object position, as in (1), while their comprehension of structures with extraction from the subject position, such as in (2), is relatively spared (Caplan & Futter, 1986; Grodzinsky, 1990; Hickok, Zurif & Canseco-Gonzalez, 1993).

(2) The boy who is kissing the girl is happy.

In contrast to English, which marks grammatical relations by word order and use of prepositions, languages with rich inflection and relatively free word order, such as Croatian, in general use case inflection to mark these relations. Interpretation of the Croatian counterpart to (1) and (2) does not depend on word order. This means that the processing of syntax in morphologically rich languages is facilitated by inflectional cues. These, however, are by definition impaired in Broca's aphasia (Caramazza & Zurif, 1976; Grodzinsky, 1984; Badecker & Caramazza, 1985; Goodglass, 1993; Caplan, 1995; Zurif, 1995). A failure to interpret a sentence may occur even when a patient's ability to process grammatical morphemes is spared. For example, Caramazza and Miceli (1991) report a dissociation between spared processing of morphological information in a sentence and impairment in thematic roles assignment in active and passive reversible sentences. The dissociation indicates a separate thematic roles processor that functions independently from other processors (Caramazza & Miceli, 1991).

Cross-linguistic research on aphasia has provided abundant evidence that manifestations of the deficit differ across languages, which is not surprising given that languages differ structurally (Grodzinsky, 1984). For example, dropping articles in speech production is typical of English-speaking Broca's aphasics. Yet this is not an option in Croatian, because this language does not have articles.

Smith and Mimica (1984) tested comprehension of semantically reversible passive sentences in 10 Serbo-Croatian[1] Broca's aphasics using the act-out testing paradigm[2]. They found that Broca's aphasics showed "some sensitivity" to case inflection, and that, when sentence comprehension was in addition facilitated by other cues (semantic cues and word position in a sentence), their aphasics' comprehension was close to that of neurologically intact control subjects. Although they used a different testing paradigm (grammaticality judgements), Lukatela, Crain and Shankweiler (1988) also found that 6 Serbo-Croatian speaking Broca's aphasics "retained sensitivity to the closed-class morphology" when sentence comprehension exclusively depended on case inflection (p. 7). Thus, Serbo-Croatian-speaking aphasics showed that they could exploit grammatical information conveyed by case inflection to different degrees, depending on the type of task. These findings challenge the claim that use of inflectional morphology is reduced in Broca's aphasics, giving rise to the claim that the deficit manifests differently in structurally different languages (Paradis, 2001).

---

[1] In this book I use the term *Serbo-Croatian* only when reporting or commenting on works that were published before the Croatian language was officially established (1991), or when referring to the works of those researchers who still use the term *Serbo-Croatian* for both Serbian and Croatian. Otherwise, I use the term *Croatian*.

[2] See section 6.2.1 on paradigms used in testing aphasic populations.

Lukatela (1989) tested comprehension of semantically reversible subject and object relative clauses formed by *koji* "which" in 7 Broca's and 5 Wernicke's Serbo-Croatian speaking aphasics. She found that Broca's performed better than Wernicke's aphasics on all types of relative clauses, and that, as with English aphasics (Caramazza & Zurif, 1976), object relative clauses were most difficult for Serbo-Croatian aphasics. However, unlike English Broca's aphasics, who comprehended object relatives at chance level, 4 out of 7 Serbo-Croatian speaking Broca's aphasics tested by Lukatela (1989) and further analysed by her and her colleagues, performed above chance on these structures (Lukatela, Shankweiler & Crain, 1995).

Thus, given the structural differences between English and Croatian, and the findings indicating that Serbo-Croatian Broca's aphasics (a) can employ inflectional cues to some extent, and (b) comprehend object relative clauses above the chance level, the question that emerges is: How do they comprehend structures where the grammatical function of the object is unambiguously signalled by case inflection on a word in sentence initial position? Such structures are direct object *who* (3) and *which NP* questions (4).

(3) Koga je lane liznulo?
"Who did the fawn lick?"
(4) Koje ždrijebe je žirafa ritnula?
"Which foal did the giraffe kick?"

In this book I explore how Croatian-speaking Broca's and patients with mixed aphasia comprehend *who* and *which NP* direct questions and other *wh*-dependencies, assuming that the processing of complex syntax requires a comprehension system that engages a network of brain areas implicated in functioning of different subsystems.

There are three main reasons for undertaking this research. First, previous studies on the comprehension of *wh*-dependencies in English-speaking agrammatic Broca's aphasics have reported contradictory findings. Hickok and Avrutin (1996) argue that Broca's aphasics display the following pattern in the comprehension of *wh*-questions:
(a) good comprehension of both subject and object direct *who* questions;
(b) good comprehension of subject, but poor comprehension of object direct *which NP* questions.

However, attempts to replicate the pattern were only partially successful: Tait, Thompson and Ballard, (1995) found that only 2 in 4, and Thomspon, Tait, Ballard and Fix (1999) showed that only 1 out of 4

Broca's aphasics followed the pattern. Salis and Edwards (2008) tested 5 English-speaking Broca's aphasics and found that the pattern of comprehension deficit in their patients did not match the pattern reported by Hickok and Avrutin. In a study with 9 German-speaking Broca's aphasics, Neuhaus and Penke (2008) found that the comprehension pattern of 3 patients did match the *who/which* pattern described above. Taken together, these findings indicate that additional crosslinguistic evidence on processing of *wh*-structures in aphasia is much needed.

Second, among the proposals that have been put forth to explain the pattern, two suggest structural explanations in terms of Universal Grammar (Hickok & Avrutin, 1996; Thompson et al.[3], 1999), implying that the pattern should exist cross-linguistically. By presenting data from a language structurally different from English, such as Croatian, this book intends to explore the cross-linguistic potential of the pattern and applicability of the proposed structural explanations.

Third, the book intends to further our understanding of computational processes involved in comprehension of complex syntax.

2.1 Computational or Conceptual Deficit?

There are two main approaches in the study of comprehension deficits in Broca's aphasia: the conceptual or structural, and the computational or processing accounts (Caplan, 1988; Frazier & Friederici, 1991; Lukatela et al., 1995). The processing theories explain the nature of the deficit in Broca's aphasics' comprehension in terms of an impaired access to knowledge (Linebarger, Schwartz & Saffran, 1983; Smith & Mimica, 1984; Caplan & Hildebrandt, 1988; Haarmann & Kolk, 1991; Lukatela et al., 1995; Tait et al, 1995; Thompson et al., 1999; Avrutin, 2000), while the structural theories explain the deficit as a loss of knowledge, either a complete (Caramazza & Zurif, 1976; Berndt & Caramazza, 1980) or partial loss of syntax (Grodzinsky, 1986; 1990; Hickok et al, 1993; Mauner, Fromkin & Cornell, 1993; Hickok & Avrutin, 1996).

The structural approach is based on the idea that damage to a component of Broca's area - such as the pars opercularis (BA 44) - wipes out part of syntax. The original localization theory, which associates specific brain areas with particular cognitive functions, assumed that Broca's area was a language area involved in speech production (see Caplan, 1995, and Goodglass, 1993, for an overview). The theory has been

[3] Thompson et al. (1999) actually present a semantic approach, but they also suggest a syntactic analysis in terms of Universal Grammar.

challenged on different grounds over time (Uttal, 2001), only to reappear recently, reinstated by researchers who argue that Broca's area is in fact the locus of a specific syntactic computation (Grodzinsky, 2000b). Since this area is typically damaged in Broca's aphasic patients, careful analyses of syntactic processing in this population were conducted in an attempt to correlate damage to component(s) of Broca's area with types of syntactic deficits.

There are two problems with this approach. First, growing evidence shows that Broca's area supports a variety of tasks not necessarily related to syntax or language in general[4]. Second, damage to Broca's area alone leads to transient disturbances, while Broca's aphasia is associated with larger, deeper lesions encompassing Broca's area (Dronkers, Pinker & Damasio, 2000). Thus, it is necessary to discern which components of syntactic processing are supported by Broca's area, and define other brain areas that also support syntactic processing.

Embick at al. (2000), for example, claim that the exclusive role of Broca's area is to regulate comprehension of specific intrasentential dependencies. Evidence from lesion studies suggests that these dependencies are related to syntactic movement, a specific process of forming complex syntactic structures, such as those in (3) and (4) (Grodzinsky, 2000b). Based on the functional Magnetic Resonance Imaging (fMRI) experiments conducted with healthy native Hebrew-speaking population, Ben-Shachar, Palti and Grodzinsky (2004) found a finer distinction in neurological areas involved in syntactic movement: both the left inferior frontal gyrus and left anterior insula are sensitive to movement operations. Friederici, Rüschemeyer, Hahne and Fiebach (2003) conducted fMRI experiments with a neurologically intact, German-speaking population and found that the anterior portion of the inferior frontal gyrus (BA 44 on the border to BA 45) and BA 47 are implicated in processing of long-distance dependencies, while "the posterior-inferior portion of BA 44, i.e., the inferior tip of the pars opercularis and deep frontal operculum on the border to ventral premotor cortex, is involved in on-line syntactic structure building processes" (p. 171). Nagai, Inui and Iwata (2010) present further evidence for the functional segregation of Broca's area. In a study with four Japanese Broca's aphasics, they found that the pars opercularis is involved in operational and the pars triangularis in semantic aspects of syntactic processing.

---

[4] Leaving aside the debate on the role of Broca's area in cognition, perception, and action (Kljajevic, 2011b), here I focus on the role of this area in syntactic processing of language.

Contrary to the representatives of the structural approach, proponents of the processing approach claim that Broca's area is not the locus of syntax *per se*. For example, Zurif (1995) claims that it houses processing resources implicated in "lexical (re)activation and its syntactic ramifications" (p. 394). In an Event Related Brain Potential (ERP) study that investigated auditory sentence comprehension in Broca's and Wernicke's aphasics, Swaab et al. (1997) found that aphasics' comprehension problems were due to an impairment of the process of integration of lexical information into the overall message representation: aphasics were slower than normal participants, and the delay in integration affected their comprehension.

Based on ERP and fMRI experiments conducted with neurologically intact native speakers of German, Fiebach, Schlesewsky and Friederici (2001, 2002) propose that Broca's area actually houses syntactic WM, assuming that a particular type of processing cost is implicated in comprehension of syntactic structures. While the findings on the involvement of Broca's area in an aspect of WM do not coincide with the evidence indicating the involvement of the mid-dorsolateral frontal cortex (BAs 46 and 9) in the verbal domain of WM (e.g., Petrides, Alivisatos, Meyer & Evans, 1993), Fiebach et al.'s (2001, 2002) view has been supported by further evidence (e.g., Felser, Clahsen & Münte, 2003; Fiebach et al., 2004).

Kennedy and Small (2002) conducted a cross-domain behavioral study in order to determine whether the WM resources required for comprehension of sentences that pose high WM demands are domain- (i.e., language-)specific. They used tasks matched for WM processing demands in language, mathematic and visuo-spatial WM contexts. Details aside, the mathematic and visuo-spatial tasks were intended to mimic processing demands of subject and object relative clauses (e.g., the brackets in a math task function as embedding within a sentence). They found that the "similarity of the sequence of demands" to the sentence processing task, and not the similarity of the cognitive domain, triggered similar WM demands and thus similar patterns of activity across the domains. Patel (2003, 2008) and Fedorenko, Patel, Cassanto, Winawer and Gibson (2009) discuss multimodal evidence for the shared syntactic integration resources hypothesis (SSIRH), according to which language and music share cognitive and neural resources, despite representing two different domains and employing different types of representations. Thus, perhaps a more plausible approach to the role of Broca's area in syntactic processing is one that applies the concept of syntax not exclusively to language, but rather assumes, like Townsend & Bever (2001), that syntax is a formal property of any activity based on computation[5].

Several fMRI studies have shown that increased sentential complexity correlates with an increase in activation of Broca's area (Just et al., 1996; Embick et al., 2000; Keller et al., 2001). If a general increase in complexity (and thus computation), rather than a specific syntactic process, is a reason for increase in activation in Broca's area, then this is further evidence that something other than syntax *per se* may be compromised in Broca's aphasic patients.

Additional evidence for this claim comes from early experiments on grammaticality judgements conducted with English speaking Broca's aphasic patients (Linebarger et al., 1983; see also Lukatela, (1989) for evidence from Serbian). The experiments have shown that grammatical knowledge in these patients was preserved, indicating that if the deficit typical for the syndrome is not in loss of knowledge of grammar, then it is probably processing that is disrupted in these patients.

This book investigates both structural and processing approaches in explaining the comprehension deficit of *wh*-dependencies in Broca's aphasia. It also examines recent research on processing of *wh*-dependencies in a population without neurological damage. By applying some of the ideas developed in research on processing of complex syntax in neurologically intact populations to comprehension deficits in aphasic patients, the book brings together research on damaged and neurologically intact brains.

The book consists of 9 chapters. Chapter 1 is a brief introduction to the topic of the study. Chapter 2 introduces theoretical concepts on aphasia that the study deals with: aphasia caused by a stroke, the syndrome approach to aphasia, with a special emphasize on Broca's aphasia, and the concept of agrammatism. Chapter 3 is a description of *wh*-dependencies in English and Croatian. Chapter 4 presents a theory within which most of the research on comprehension of syntax in Broca's aphasia has been conducted by now: the Government and Binding theory (Chomsky, 1981), and a theoretical account of the differences between *who* and *which NP* types of questions. This chapter also presents the general pattern and the *who/which NP* pattern of syntactic comprehension deficit in Broca's aphasia, as well as proposed structural explanations. The main topic of Chapter 5 is the processing cost of comprehension of *wh*-dependencies. Chapter 6 summarizes the research questions, introduces the hypothesis of

---

[5] "Syntax is not a unique formal property of linguistic computation, but it is part of vision, motor behavior, and every other activity with a computational basis" (Townsend & Bever, 2001, p. 1).

the present study, describes the evaluative and experimental measures and the procedures used, and briefly introduces the participants. Chapter 7 consists of eight case studies. Each case study contains information on lesion site and type of stroke in a particular patient, description of his/her spontaneous speech as well as the results of his/her performance on evaluative and experimental measures. Abstracting away from the comprehension problems of individual patients reported in Chapter 7, Chapter 8 analyzes them in terms of syntax and processing, directing the general discussion towards the implications of the findings of this study and research on language disorders for our understanding of language and cognition. Chapter 9 concludes the book by placing the gained insights in a wider theoretical context.

CHAPTER TWO

BROCA'S APHASIA

2.1 Aphasia Caused by Stroke

Aphasia is a language disorder caused by brain damage. The defining factors of aphasia are location of lesion and etiology (Benson & Ardila, 1996). Regardless of whether aphasia is caused by a vascular, traumatic, infectious, or surgical cause, its symptoms always reflect language impairment (Darley, 1982).

Most research on aphasia so far has focused on post-stroke aphasia. Stroke is among the leading causes of disability worldwide. It is also the most common cause of aphasia (Tonkonogy, 1986), which, according to some authors, leaves 20–25% of patients initially aphasic (Reinvang, 1985), while others claim that 40% of all strokes result in this disorder (Gazanniga, Ivry & Mangun, 1998).

Stroke or cerebrovascular incident is a sudden loss of circulation to an area of the brain, which causes loss or impairment of function performed by that brain area (Caplan, 2000). Two major types of stroke are ischemia and hemorrhage. In general, 80% of all strokes are categorized as acute ischemic stroke. Ischemia occurs when the blood flow to the brain tissue is either disrupted due to an occlusion of one or more blood vessels (thrombosis and embolic stroke), or is diminished due to low systemic perfusion pressure (decreased systemic perfusion). Hemorrhage is blood leakage into the brain (intracerebral hemorrhage) or into the spaces around the brain (subarachnoid hemorrhage). Stroke lesions are typically large and affect more than a single brain area, causing impairment in more than one language modality in many cases.

2.2 Classification of Aphasias

A failure of specific components of the cerebrovascular system can affect functioning of different parts of the brain. Language functioning is affected differently by damage to different parts of the brain due to stroke.

Several types of aphasia have been defined based on this neurological approach: Broca's, Wernicke's, transcortical motor aphasia, transcortical sensory aphasia, conduction, global, and anomic aphasia. There are over 20 different classifications of aphasias (Ardila, 2010), but this anatomically based syndrome typology is most dominant (Goodglass, 1993; Caplan, 1995; Basso, 2003). It classifies aphasias according to whether they result from disturbances of cortical centers (i.e., Broca's aphasia is caused by damage to Broca's area, Wernicke's aphasia results from damage to Wernicke's area) or from disruptions of connections between the centers (e.g., conduction aphasia is caused by disruption of the arcuate fasciculus) (Caplan, 1995).

This type of aphasia classification has been criticized on several grounds. For instance:

a) Goodglass (1993) and Caplan (1995) have pointed out that syndromes are too rigid to capture fuzzy areas between different types of aphasia. The clear-cut distinctions among language deficits associated with different syndromes do not reflect clinical reality (Caplan, 1995; Goodglass, 1993). For instance, a patient who is capable of producing only one-word utterances and has impaired articulation and relatively impaired comprehension, and a patient who has normal articulation but agrammatic speech output and good comprehension, are both qualified as Broca's aphasics (Goodglass, 1993).
b) The syndromes are too wide and too narrow at the same time. For example, overlapping features characterize separate syndromes: phonemic (i.e., literal) paraphasias, i.e., faulty selection of sounds, are present in Wernicke's, conduction, and global aphasias, while anomia characterizes all aphasias. However, a patient exhibiting only phonemic paraphasias and anomia cannot be classified according to this typology and as a result many cases with mixed symptoms are unclassifiable (Caplan, 1995).
c) The syndrome approach relies heavily on anatomical criteria, although they are inconsistent. For example, as Goodglass (1993) pointed out, it is not clear how to classify a disorder with characteristics of Wernicke's speech in a patient without a lesion in the temporal lobe. Similarly, different types of aphasia can follow damage to the same brain area. As an example, researchers who studied aphasia secondary to lesion of the basal ganglia, more specifically striatocapsular infarction (infarction of the head of the caudate nucleus, the putamen, and the anterior limb of the internal capsule), found that this lesion site is associated with Broca's, transcortical motor, Wernicke's,

conduction, global and anomic aphasia, or with no aphasia at all (Nadeu & Crosson, 1997).

d) The syndrome approach is incoherent with regard to the criteria it applies in classification. It mixes criteria from different domains: a certain type of aphasia is classified as such based on the type of channels that are involved (e.g., sensory vs. motor channels), the type of produced linguistic errors (e.g., agrammatism, paraphasias anomia) and impressions of fluency (fluent vs. non-fluent) (Goodglass, 1993).
e) The syndrome approach describes types of aphasia as "fixed patterns of linguistic behaviour", despite possible differences in language performance due to severity of aphasia and individual differences (Goodglass, 1993).
f) The classical syndrome approach to aphasia cannot capture the intra- and inter-individual differences (Goodglass, 1993; Murray, 1999). As an example, Bastiaanse (1995) reports on a patient who shifted between short, well-formed sentences and agrammatic speech during a single interview.
g) The syndrome approach also assumes that language is a set of activities such as naming, writing, reading, speaking (Grodzinsky, 2000b). From the linguistic point of view, this means that the syndrome approach fails to recognize language as a system of knowledge organized into subsystems (modules) that can be selectively disrupted depending on the brain damage. In the linguistic literature, this knowledge has been referred to as *linguistic competence*, as opposed to *linguistic performance*, i.e., actual use of language (Chomsky, 1981). By failing to recognize this distinction, the classical syndrome approach falls behind the recent insights on language.

Some researchers have pointed out that the cause of the problem with the classification of aphasias is the concept of syndrome itself (Berndt & Caramazza, 1980), while others have emphasized the lack of consensus on how to classify the various manifestations of aphasia (Caplan, 1995; Goodglass, 1993). Another view emphasizes that after a brain injury, behaviour results from the functioning of the entire brain, and symptoms are therefore "not manifestations of the injured brain region, rather they are expression of plastic changes in the rest of the brain" (Pascual-Leone, Amedi, Fregni & Marabet, 2005).

Few workable alternatives to the classical syndrome approach have been formulated. One possibility is a cognitive approach to language disorders, i.e., search for the underlying cause of a deficit, and its interpretation in terms of modularity (or differently interpreted functional organization of cognition). The modular approach is based on the idea that the functional architecture of cognition is organized in such a way that language processing is carried out by processing modules (components) that are presumably common to and arranged in the same way in all language users. As a focal brain injury, aphasia can disrupt functioning of a specific component of the normal functional architecture, sparing other components. Thus, the cognitive approach to aphasia has advantages over the syndromic approach in relating functioning of damaged and neurologically intact brains. However, this approach seems to leave open the question of how to best classify aphasic patients.

Another option is a clinical nonsyndromic approach, which briefly describes a particular case of aphasia as a cluster of symptoms, capturing at the same time all the details of a specific case (Goodglass, 1993). The advantage of this approach over the classic syndromic approach is that it allows occurrence of both prototypical and borderline cases without forcing the mixed cases into "pure" syndromes.

If genuine explanations explain phenomena in a principled way, then in the case of language such an explanation would link normal language processing with its furthest poles in both directions: language acquisition and language disorders. Assuming that aphasics' language is essentially different from language produced by a neurologically intact brain, the syndrome approach has missed linking the three domains.

Until recently, most of the research on aphasia neglected the fact that other sources of information (e.g., visual) are present simultaneously with language information, and that other types of cognitive resources (e.g., memory, attention) are engaged in language processing. For example, although critical in syntactic processing, the role of WM in aphasic language processing has begun to be investigated only recently. Research on aphasia and attention is also sparse, although it is reasonable to assume with Murray (1999) that the within-subject variability is probably caused by attention deficits typically present in aphasic patients.

Instead of approaching aphasia as an isolated cognitive accident manifested as language disturbance of a type that depends on lesion site, and given the lack of typology that overcomes the drawbacks of the dominant approach discussed above, in this book I consider all the symptoms of a particular case available from the medical documentation, whether they fit into the classic definition of the syndrome or not, as well as all the available characteristics of that person's speech and comprehension as revealed by the evaluative and experimental measures (see Chapter 7).

2.3 Broca's Aphasia from a Neuroanatomical Perspective

One common traditional definition of Broca's aphasia assumes a language disorder due to a lesion in Broca's area, which has been described as a *classical language area* implicated in speech production. However, this view has been challenged due to growing evidence indicating that Broca's area contributes not only to speech, but also to other aspects of language, supporting tasks unrelated to language as well, such as memory tasks, action observation, mental imagery of movement, musical syntax, processing of complex geometric patterns, and so on. These findings indicate that some traditional assumptions on Broca's area do not hold[1]. Furthermore, Broca's aphasia has been associated with lesions in other brain areas, and it has also been shown that lesion in the left inferior frontal gyrus (LIFG) alone does not cause the classical Broca's aphasia. A revised notion of lesion causing the syndrome includes some combination of the LIFG with other brain areas. Depending on this combination, three distinct subtypes of Broca's aphasia are now discernible (Alexander, Naeser & Palumbo, 1990).

2.3.1 From *Circonvolution du Langage* to Broca's Area

In a recent metaanalysis of 542 articles containing the term Broca's area/region, published between 1994 and 2004, Lindenberg, Fangerau and Seitz (2007) found that the term Broca's area was not defined in 21% of these papers. Of those that defined the term, 97% of papers specified it anatomically (either cytoarchitectonically or macroscopically) and 3% determined it functionally. However, Broca's area as an anatomical concept is heterogeneous: when determined cytoarchitectonically in terms of BAs, it is consistently defined as BAs 44 and 45 in only 27% of papers, while in the rest of papers the term refers to BA 44 in some papers and includes (some combination of) BAs 44, 45, 47, 46, and 6, in others. In addition, descriptive terms such as a *Broca's area proper* or *restricted Broca's area,* on one side, and an *extended Broca's area, Broca's region, Broca's complex, Broca's area as a large area*, on the other, are also in use. Furthermore, the area is often described in terms of gyral patterns and sulcal landmarks, even though the boundaries of the macroscopic landmarks do not always coincide with the microscopic boundaries (Amunts, Schleicher, Bürgel, Mohlberg, Uylings & Zilles, 1999).

---

[1] Parts of Section 2.3 appeared in my paper *Broca's Area: Four Misconceptions,* in: *Current Topics in Neurology, Psychiatry and Related Disciplines, 19(1)*, 20-30.

Functional and neuroanatomical heterogeneity of other language areas, such as Wernicke's, have also been demonstrated (Wise, Scott, Blank, Mummery, Murphy & Warburton, 2001). For instance, damage to the fronto-temporal region of Wernicke's area has been associated with lexical processing impairment, while damage to the parietal-temporal region of this area has been associated with a syntactic processing deficit (Caramazza & Zurif, 1976). This evidence further highlights the need to re-examine the neuroanatomical classification of aphasia.

Broca's area is a complex concept that has become associated with a loss of speech in two patients described by Pierre Paul Broca in the 1860s. Its status as a *classical language area* supporting speech production, or *the motor center for speech*, had remained intact for more than 100 years, only to become challenged in light of neuroimaging evidence. Neuroanatomically, the area was associated with the site of lesion that allegedly caused the loss of speech in Broca's patients Leborgne and Lelong—the LIFG.

The development of the term from *circonvolution du langage* to *Broca's area* began in the 1860s, when Broca reported that his two now famous patients, Leborgne and Lelong, who exhibited a profound speech loss, had damage to the inferior frontal gyrus of the left brain hemisphere. Broca hypothesized that this brain area was responsible for speech production and named the disorder *aphemia* (Greek a "without", phemia "speech"), intending to convey the idea that the disorder had spared the language faculty, selectively affecting only the faculty of speech. At autopsy Broca found that for instance Leborgne's lesion was much larger, affecting in addition to the posterior half of the inferior frontal gyrus, the middle frontal gyrus, insula, and the striate body (Broca, 1861/2001). Broca argued that Leborgne's lesion had been progressive, originating probably at the IFG, spreading over the frontal gyri, and eventually reaching the insula and the striate body. As a consequence, in addition to speech loss, which had characterized the first ten years of his illness, Leborgne had experienced a general cognitive decline, and the right limbs' paralysis during the last eleven years of his life.

The brains of Leborgne and Lelong, which have been preserved and kept in the Musee Dupuytren in Paris, France, were recently inspected by the techniques such as computerized tomography (CT) and magnetic resonance imaging (MRI). These techniques revealed that Leborgne's lesion in the frontal lobe was in the middle third, not in the posterior third, of the inferior frontal gyrus (Dronkers, Plaisant, Iba-Zizen & Cabanis, 2007), affecting entire insula and the basal ganglia, while Lelong's lesion affected half of the pars opercularis in the posterior, inferior frontal gyrus (BA 44), while sparing the pars triangularis (BA 45). In addition, both patients had damage to the arcuate/superior longitudinal fasciculus. Thus, both brains had lesions that are inconsistent with the current concept of Broca's area, which is restricted to the posterior third of the LIFG. More importantly, they both had damage to the arcuate/superior longitudinal fasciculus, which seems to be a more likely cause of the profound, long-lasting speech production deficit in these two patients (Dronkers et al., 2007).

2.3.2 Is Broca's Area an Anatomical Area Per Se?

Despite the general lack of consensus on what constitutes Broca's area (Lindenberg et al., 2007), there is some agreement among researchers that this area is neuroanatomically associated with the pars opercularis (BA 44) and pars triangularis (BA 45) of the LIFG (Greenlee, Oya, Kawasaki, Volkov & Severson, 2007). Both the gross structure and the cytoarchitectonics of the LIFG are marked by interindividual variability. In addition, the two brain areas differ in their postnatal trajectories and there is evidence on differences in their respective functionalities. This has led some authors to conclude that Broca's area is not an anatomical area per se (e.g., Hagoort, 2005).

Individual differences in the brain's organization of language have been recognized at several levels: "in the gross anatomy of human left perisylvian cortex, … in the gyral pattern at the end of the sylvian fissure…, in the extent of the planum temporale … and in the extent of its specific cytoarchitectonic areas…" (Ojemann, 1991, p. 2283). Amunts and Zilles (2006) also point out the individual variability in cytoarchitectonic features. As an example, in a study by Amunts and her colleagues (1999) it was shown that volumes of BAs 44 and 45 differed in 20 post-mortem brains by a factor of 10, which is much larger when compared to interindividual differences found in other brain regions (*cf.* the hyppocampi volume in the same post-mortem brains differed only by a factor of 2).

Applying a quantitative and observer-independent cytoarchitectonic analysis of BAs 44 and 45, Amunts et al. (1999) found that BA 44 and BA 45 differed in granularity in layer IV: area 44 had "a barely recognizable dysgranular layer IV" (p. 325). More specifically, layer IV was visible, but it could not appear as a layer containing the granular cells exclusively, because it was invaded to different degrees by the pyramidal cells from the lower part of layer III and from the upper part of layer V. On the contrary, BA 45 "differed essentially from area 44 by the presence of a clearly visible layer IV" (*ibid*). Other differences between BAs 44 and 45 include left-larger-than-right volume of BA 44, but not of BA 45 (Amunts & Zilles, 2006), and a significant left-over-right asymmetry in cell density for BA 44, but not for BA 45 in adult brains (Amunts et al., 1999).

Furthermore, distinct postnatal developmental trajectories were also reported for BA 44 and BA 45. A study of 34 human brains has shown that asymmetry between the left and right BAs 44 and 45, which was established by the age of 1, tended to increase with age, reaching an adult-like asymmetry at the age of 5 in BA 45 and at the age of 11 in BA 44 (Amunts, Schleicher, Ditterich & Zilles, 2003).

Although the exact functional differences between BA 44 and BA 45 are still not known (Greenlee et al, 2007), the cytoarchitectonic differences between the pars opercularis and pars triangularis of the LIFG indicate that these areas' respective functionalities may differ to a greater extent than previously assumed. Amunts, Schleicher and Zilles (2004) compared the cytoarchitecture of BAs 44 and 45 of Mr. Emil Krebs, who spoke fluently more than 60 languages, with the cytoarchitecture of the same brain areas in 11 male control brains. They found statistically significant cytoarchitectonic differences between Krebs' and controls' left and right BA 44, and in right BA 45, while no significant difference was found when the cytoarchitecture of visual area BA 18 was compared between E.K.'s and the controls' brains. Thus, there is a relationship between the cytoarchitecture of BAs 44, 45 and language abilities.

2.3.3 Broca's Area is Not Dedicated Exclusively to Language

Following early work of Broca, the involvement of the LIFG in speech production has been confirmed by the evidence from numerous lesion studies associated with aphasia, and recently by neuroimaging evidence on neurologically intact populations (Hillis, 2007). Whereas Broca's area supports speech production, nonfluent speech may also result from a disconnection of Broca's area from the superior temporal cortex and damage to the insular white matter (Bonilha & Fridriksson, 2009).

The assumption that Broca's area is an exclusive motor center for speech has been challenged since the 1970s (Caramazza & Zurif, 1976; Mohr, 1976), due to the evidence on this area's involvement in comprehension of complex syntactic structures. Furthermore, a growing body of neuroimaging evidence suggests that this area is involved not only in syntax (Just et al., 1996; Stromswold et al., 1996; Caplan et al., 2000; Embick et al., 2000; Sakai, Noguchi, Takeuchi & Watanabe, 2002; Ben-Shachar et al., 2004), including artificial languages (Peterson, Forkstam & Ingvar, 2004), but also in language tasks that are not of syntactic nature, such as phonological and semantic processing (Poldrack et al., 1999, 2001; Price, 1998), and in language-related memory tasks (Kaan & Stowe, 2002; Baldo & Dronkers, 2006). It is also involved in language unrelated tasks, such as processing of complex geometric patterns (Fink et al., 2006), music (Maess, Koelsch, Gunter & Friederici, 2001), grasping movement/manipulation and mental imagery of grasping (Binkofski & Buccino, 2004; Decety et al., 1994), in observation of meaningful but not meaningless hand actions (Fadiga & Craighero, 2006), motor imagery (Binkofski et al., 2001; Decety & Grèzes, 2006), and so on. Thus, an impressive body of neuroimaging evidence on Broca's area's involvement in a variety of cognitive, perceptual, and motor tasks indicates that this brain area is neither specialized exclusively for speech or syntax, nor dedicated exclusively to language.

Several proposals attempting to explain the functionality of Broca's area have been put forth. For instance, Thompson-Schill (2005) proposes that Broca's area supports selection of information from competing sources. Novick, Trueswell and Thompson-Schill (2005, 2010) argue that Broca's area serves a broader cognitive control function. Greewe, Bornkessel, Zysset, Wiese, von Cramon and Schlesewsky (2005) present evidence that indicates involvement of BA 44 in language specific linearization of hierarchical language dependencies, and Opitz and Friederici (2007) provide further support to this finding, claiming that this area's involvement in the processing of hierarchical dependencies may not be unique to language, but perhaps also found in imitation and musical syntax. In conclusion, lesion studies and recent neuroimaging evidence indicate that Broca's area is associated not only with speech (as a motor function), but also with other language and non-language tasks involving other aspects of cognition, verbal WM, selection processes, and so on.

2.3.4 Broca's Area-Broca's Aphasia

The traditional notion that Broca's aphasia is caused by damage to the LIFG has been challenged on several grounds. First, damage to the posterior part of the IFG causes only mild, transient speech problems that do not qualify as Broca's aphasia (Dronkers et al., 2000). Lesions typically associated with Broca's aphasia are larger, involving adjacent cortical and underlying subcortical areas that subserve different functions, because strokes typically affect multiple areas (Alexander et al., 1990). For instance, they may include the immediate premotor and motor regions, and the underlying white matter, the basal ganglia, and the insula (Damasio, 1991; Ardila, 2010). Second, cases of Broca's aphasia without damage to

Broca's area were reported (e.g., Dronkers, Wilkins, Van Valin, Redfern & Jaeger, 1994). Third, damage to this region was reported to also cause *fluent* aphasia with impairment of syntactic comprehension (Mohr, 1976; Alexander et al., 1990). It appears then that damage to Broca's area is neither sufficient nor necessary to induce Broca's aphasia.

2.4 Broca's Aphasia from a Linguistic Perspective

As described by Paul Broca, the most prominent symptom of the language disorder that became known later as Broca's aphasia is related to language production:

> […] what is missing in these patients is only the faculty to articulate words; they hear and understand all that is said to them, they have all their intelligence and they emit easily vocal sounds.

It is manifested as laboured and distorted articulation:

> They execute with their tongue and their lips movements larger and more energetic than would be necessary to articulate sounds, and nonetheless, the well-sensed response which they would like to make, becomes reduced to a very small number of articulate sounds (Broca, 1861/ 2001).

Broca was right in pointing out the articulatory problem in these patients. Indeed, articulation disturbances in these patients can be anywhere from mild to severe, and when they are more pronounced, speech is halted, forced. The disorder is often accompanied by buccofacial apraxia as well as by right hemiparesis and ideomotor apraxia of the right arm (Spreen & Risser, 2003; Basso, 2003). In addition, semantic and phonemic paraphasias, impoverished use of verbs, difficulty with function words (so-called telegraphic speech) and reduced sentence length and complexity also characterize speech output of Broca's aphasics (Alexander et al., 1990).

However, contrary to Broca's observations, comprehension in these patients also varies. Generally, they comprehend words better than sentences. The syntactic impairment, which also varies from patient to patient, runs cross-modally and is reflected in auditory comprehension and reading, and, as some researchers claim (Berndt & Caramazza, 1980), in metalinguistic abilities (Linebarger et al., 1983, argue for the opposite claim). Sentence comprehension is in particular impaired when it depends on syntax. A dominant view on this type of aphasia today is that Broca's aphasics have difficulty following the rules of grammar, both in speech production and comprehension (Goodglass, 1993), but not necessarily to the same extent.

2.4.1 Agrammatism

A broad definition of agrammatism assumes a sensitivity to grammar at all levels (word, phrase, sentence and discourse) in both language production and comprehension. Grammar-related deficits had been reported in early research on Broca's aphasia. For example, J.J. Wepfer's *The Medical-Practical Observations of Effects Inside and Outside the Head*, written in the 17th century, refers to a patient who "had suddenly forgotten all names", including his own (anomia). From time to time, he would also "violate syntactic rules and, contrary to the structure of German sentences, he would prepose one word to another and sometimes he could not complete a word" (cited in Whitaker, 1997, p. 2). However, the early research on agrammatism had focused on speech production, i.e., on expressive aspects of agrammatism, emphasizing the omission of grammatical morphemes, which include function words (e.g., articles, conjunctions) and inflectional endings (morphemes marking morphological case, subject-verb agreement, verb tense etc.)[2] (Whitaker, 1997; Goodglass, 1993). While the proponents of the so-called classical research on aphasia (Broca, Wernicke, Lichteim, Dejerine, Marie) were mostly interested in word-level phenomena in aphasia, the proponents of premodern work on agrammatism (Head, Jackson, Pick) focused on syntax.

For instance, Pick's monograph published at the beginning of the 20th century contains observations on some patients' impairment of specific aspects of sentence comprehension even though their word comprehension was preserved. Pick developed a model of agrammatism which allowed selective disruption of syntactic components in Broca's patients (Whitaker, 1997). However, his ideas on syntactic disturbances in aphasia did not have impact on the field at that time and the view of Broca's aphasia as a pure speech deficit prevailed till the early 1970s.

The observation that Broca's aphasic patients have difficulty understanding sentences in which meaning depends exclusively on syntactic information reappeared with Caramazza and Zurif (1976), who argued for a cross-modally symmetric deficit in these patients. The idea of

---

[2] Substitutions of grammatical elements, on the other side, characterize Wernicke's aphasia by definition. However, in some languages (e.g., Slavic) Broca's aphasics also substitute grammatical elements.

a central syntactic deficit underlying agrammatism in Broca's aphasia was further elaborated into the overarching agrammatism hypothesis (OAA).

Since OAA postulates a parallelism in speech and comprehension patterns in Broca's aphasics (Caramazza & Zurif, 1976), it was claimed that syntax of these patients was limited not only in production, but also in comprehension (Kean, 1984). However, the collected evidence suggests that many Broca's agrammatic aphasics with poor speech production can have well preserved comprehension (Swinney & Zurif, 1993). Another important implication of OAA is that Broca's area is involved not only in speech production, but also in speech comprehension, which subsequent research has confirmed. OAA turned out to be a too strong hypothesis, although some researchers still claim that a viable option of OAA is possible (Grodzinsky, 2000a). In retrospect, the main contribution of this hypothesis probably consists in drawing attention to comprehension patterns in Broca's aphasia.

Caramazza and Zurif (1976) proposed that breakdown in syntactic comprehension in Broca's aphasics—asyntactic comprehension—resulted from a loss of control over the "algorithmic processes" (i.e., grammar). Asyntactic comprehension refers to impairment in comprehension of semantically reversible sentences (due to inability to correctly assign thematic roles) in a patient who understands non-reversible sentences, and words (Druks & Marshall, 1995). Interestingly, asyntactic comprehension seems to follow rules of grammar (Berndt & Caramazza, 1980).

Adherence to the rules of grammar was also recognized in the patterns of Broca's aphasics' speech production deficit. For instance, Heeschen and Kolk (1988) found that German-speaking agrammatics omitted inflection of finite verbs, while following the rule on verb position in a sentence:

> ...if there was just omission of inflection, a sentence like *X trinkt gerne Bier* would lead to the ungrammatical *X trinken gerne Bier*. However, the aphasic omitters indeed shift the verb to the end so that a grammatically correct word order results: *X gerne Bier trinken* (Heeschen & Kolk, 1988, p. 300).

Ulatowska et al. (2001) report on a Polish Broca's aphasic patient who developed a strategy of substituting the locative suffix *–ie*, which requires a stem alternation involving palatalization, by another *locative* suffix, *-u*, which does not require the stem alternation. For example, the patient would say *polityk głosi o kryzysu*$_{\text{Loc.sg.f.}}$, instead of saying *polityk głosi o kryzysie*$_{\text{Loc.sg.m.}}$, "The politician talks about the crisis" (Ulatowska et al., 2001; p. 328). Thus, although the patient made a substitution error, she also followed the rule requiring that a noun in the locative case follow the preposition *o*.

If Broca's aphasics still follow the rules of grammar in speech production in spite of its breakdown, do they follow the rules of grammar in comprehension when it is impaired? The current linguistic research on aphasia is focused on finding out evidence for a breakdown of these rules in Broca's aphasia. This book investigates whether the set of rules employed in formation of structures with *who* and *which NP*, that has been claimed to cause difficulty comprehending these structures in English-speaking aphasics, is disrupted in Croatian-speaking aphasic patients.

CHAPTER THREE

DESCRIPTION OF *WH*-DEPENDENCIES

3.1 *Who* and *Which NP* as Indicators of *Wh*-Dependencies

Wh-dependencies are dependency relations that hold between a *wh*-word, such as *who, what, why, when, which, how* ("in *what* way"), and another element in a sentence. A dependency relation in syntax is determined by the identity of elements that enter it, as well as by the distance between them, which in turn is determined by their syntactic hierarchy. Since English has a fixed word order, it marks grammatical relations between *wh*-words such as *who/which NP* and the rest of the sentence by the order of words. *Who* in (1) and *which camel* in (2) are both objects indicated by the presence of the subjects *the fawn* and *the zebra* before the verb.

(1) Who did the fawn lick?
(2) Which camel did the zebra kick?

There are syntactic, semantic, and discourse constraints on the distribution of *who/which NP* in English. Syntactic constraints regulate sentential hierarchy and dependency relations. For example, they require that sentences such as (1) and (2) always have a *wh*-word at the very beginning of the sentence. In a case such as (3), which contains two *wh*-words, syntactic constraints require that *who* appear in the sentence-initial position, and *which book* in the sentence final position. Any violation of this requirement results in a grammatically incorrect sentence, such as (4).

(3) Who read which book?
(4) *Which book read who?

Semantically, *who* is more general and as such has a wider distribution than *which NP*. Namely, *who* can appear in any context, grammatically tied up with nouns in singular as well as plural, referring to one or more entities in the discourse. However, *which NP* is allowed only in a sentence that presupposes the existence of a set of entities. Thus, it would be odd to ask *Which fawn licked the frog* in a context where there is only one fawn. In that sense, *who* is semantically indeterminate and more open than *which NP*. Another semantic difference between the two pertains to animacy. The interrogative-relative pronoun *who* is restricted to animate things; *which NP* can be used for both animate and inanimate things.

Unlike English, Croatian is a morphologically rich language with relatively free word order, and as such it offers an excellent opportunity to manipulate sentential dependencies and thereby test differences in comprehension of *wh*-constructions with different degrees of complexity. Among other forms, Croatian uses interrogative-relative pronoun *tko* ("who") and adjectival pronoun *koji, koja, koje* ("which") to form *wh*-dependencies in structures such as direct and embedded questions, and relative clauses. *Wh*-words such as *tko,* and *koji, koja, koje* are informationally multilevel, because they bring in three types of information: morphological, syntactic and semantic. Morphologically, *tko* is less informative than *koji, koja, koje*: the former carries information on case only, and not on gender and number, while the pronouns *koji, koja, koje*, in addition to case, carry information on gender and number.

Table 3-1: Morphological information contained in *tko* and *koji*.

Morphological information	Case	Gender	Number
tko "who"	+	-	-
koji, koja, koje "which"	+	+	+

Syntactically, *tko* behaves differently from *koji, koja, koje* (see Chapter 4). The morphological information contained in the pronouns above and the syntactic information in the rest of the sentence build up a syntactic representation, while semantic information, mostly determined by the meaning of the clausal verb, is used to build the propositional representation (Noordman & Vonk, 1999). Semantically, *koji, koja, koje* are reduced to a set of potential referents by discourse, as in English, and thus they are more determined than *tko.*

Croatian also uses prosodic features to distinguish between the interrogative-relative pronoun *tko* and the adjectival pronoun *koji,* as shown in Brabec, Hraste & Živković's (1958) examples presented here as (5) and (6): kòmu (who_{Dat}) is a Dative form of *tko* and is used for a referent that has not yet been mentioned in the discourse, while *kômu/kôm* is a

Dative form of *koji* "which" and is used for referring to something that has already been introduced in the discourse.

(5) Kòmu (*tko*) si pozajmio knjigu?
"Whom$_{Dat}$ did you lend the book to?"
(6) Učenik kômu/kôm (*koji*) si posudio knjigu neka je vrati.
"The student to whom$_{Dat}$ you lent the book should return it."

Tko and *koji* differ in the oblique cases listed below only in the quantity and length of accent (Brabec et al., 1958, p. 98):

Tko: Genitive: kòga (kog); Dative/Locative: kòmu (kom)
Koji: Genitive: kôga (kôg); Dative/Locative: kômu (kôm)

(7) Ò kom (*tko*) to govoriš?
"Who$_{Loc}$ are you talking about?"
(8) Čovjek o kôm$_{Loc}$ (*koji*) govoriš je moj prijatelj.
"The man you are talking about is a friend of mine."

The Accusative form of the pronoun *kòji* for masculine inanimate things is identical to the form of Nominative. When *koji* refers to animate masculine things, its Accusative form differs in type and length of accent from the Accusative form of the pronoun *tko*:

(9) Ne znam kòga (*tko*) bih poslao po knjigu.
"I don't know who to send to pick up the book."
(10) Učenik, kôga$_{Acc}$ (*koji*) sam posalo po knjigu, vratio se.
"The student I sent to pick up the book has returned."

Finally, *koji, koja, koje* can convey three different types of meaning - relative, interrogative and indeterminate, as pointed out by Kordić (1995) and shown in (11a-c).

(11) a. Ne znam dijete *koje* pjeva.
"I do not know the child who is singing."
b. *Koje* dijete pjeva?
"Which child is singing?"
c. Moglo bi *koje* zapjevati.
"A child could sing."

In other words, there is nothing inherent to *koji, koja, koje* that indicates that it should be interpreted as a relative, indeterminate or an interrogative word: these meanings are imposed on it by discourse. This is not language-specific. For example, the meaning of the Japanese *wh*-word *dare* is potentially interrogative, existential, and universal, so that the discourse determines its interpretation (Cheng, 1997).

3.2 *Wh*-Dependencies in English

Syntactic structures that contain *wh*-dependencies are: direct questions as in (12), embedded questions as in (13), sentences with relative clauses as in (14), cleft sentences as in (15), and pseudo-clefts as in (16). Yes/no questions do not belong to *wh*-dependencies, because the auxiliary *do* is not a *wh*-word[1]

(12) Who did the fawn lick?
(13) I wonder who the fawn licked.
(14) The frog who the fawn licked jumped into water.
(15) It was the frog that the fawn licked.
(16) The one who the fawn licked was the frog.

All grammars, including both traditional grammar (i.e., pre-generative and pre-Chomskyan syntax) as well as generative grammar, assume that sentences (12)–(16) above are derived from a basic structure like (17).

(17) The fawn licked the frog.

The arguments for this claim are based on three pieces of evidence (Brown & Miller, 1991):

- Frequency - the basic structure is more frequent than the derived structure;
- Adjacency - the related constituents of the basic structure are adjacent, not separated by other constituents;
- Sufficiency - the basic structure does not require insertion of additional syntactic elements.

As we will see in Chapter 4, generative grammar offers other evidence for this claim.

---

[1] Yes/no questions and less frequent *wh*-structures, such as echo questions (e.g., *He saw what!*) and *wh*-exclamations (e.g., *What fun we had!*), are not the focus of the present discussion.

3.2.1 Direct *Wh*-Questions

Direct *wh*-questions are questions formed by *wh*-words, as in (18) and (19).

(18) *Who* chased the zebra?
(19) *Who* did the tiger chase?

The term *wh-questions* can be misleading, because ***wh**ether* questions also begin with *wh-*, but they are not *wh*-questions; at the same time, *how*, which does not have the *wh*-marker, actually is a *wh*-question (Karttunen, 1978). Still, *wh-* has become a marker of *wh*-words, adopted in analyses of other languages in which these words do not contain a *wh*-element phonetically.

Traditional grammar suggests that direct questions such as (18) and (19) are formed from a declarative sentence (20), by replacing a noun with an interrogative pronoun (e.g., *wh*-words such as *who*, *what*):

(20) The tiger chased the zebra.

The interrogative pronoun thus takes the sentence initial position and is immediately followed by the auxiliary (Brown & Miller, 1991). The traditional syntactic analysis of interrogative sentences introduced by *wh*-words disregards the nature of the dependency relations, such as those defined by Chomskyan grammar (Chomsky, 1975, 1981), or the distance between a moved element and its original position, explaining the difference between (18) and (19) only in terms of grammatical function: the former is a subject question, while the latter is an object question.

Direct questions can be spread across more than one clause, as in (21) and (22), where the *wh*-word originates in the embedded clause and moves to the beginning of the matrix clause.

(21) Who do you think chased the zebra?
(22) Which giraffe do you think the fawn followed?

Apart from single (matrix) questions, there are multiple questions such as (23), which involve more than one *wh*-word:

(23) Who chased whom?

Finally, direct questions can be passivized, like in (24) and (25).

(24) Who was chased by the tiger?
(25) Which zebra was the giraffe followed by?

3.2.2 Embedded *Wh*-Questions

Direct questions, both single (18), (19), and multiple (23) can be embedded as in (26)-(28).

(26) I wonder who chased the zebra.
(27) I know who the tiger chased.
(28) I forgot who chased who.

When they are embedded within another sentence, direct questions are referred to as indirect or embedded questions[2]. Syntactically, the embedding process changes the status of a question from matrix to subordinate, although the syntactic hierarchy and grammatical functions within the embedded question remain unchanged, due to the fact that the auxiliary does not change its position. Semantically, apart from the general constraints on the distribution of *wh*-words determined by the nature of the antecedent (e.g., *who* refers to animate and *what* to inanimate objects), the distribution and meaning of embedded questions depend on verbs that require this kind of embedding. There are many semantic categories of question embedding verbs, such as verbs of retaining and acquiring knowledge, verbs of communication, decision verbs, inquisitive verbs, and so on (Karttunen, 1978). Thus, with respect to the type of clause they form, questions can be direct or embedded; with respect to the number of *wh*-words they contain, questions can be single or multiple.

3.2.3 Relative Clauses

Generally, relative clauses are subordinate clauses in complex sentences that modify a noun phrase of the main clause (de Rijk, 1972). In (29) the relative clause is shown in italics, and the noun phrase it modifies is underlined.

(29) The lion *who kicked the zebra* fell asleep.

---

[2] Since the term *indirect questions* has been used in the literature with different meanings, as pointed out by Hausser (1983), which can be misleading, I use the term *embedded questions*.

The relative clause in (29) modifies its antecedent in the sense that it conveys some information about the referent of that antecedent. Depending on the way information is conveyed, relative clauses are divided into restrictive and non-restrictive relative clauses. A restrictive relative clause cannot be omitted without a change in a sentence meaning (*The only person who can help me now is my mother*), while the non-restrictive relative clauses can be omitted from the sentence without any change in meaning (*The book, which I am reading so carefully, is about syntax*). Thus, an antecedent refers to something, and a relative clause modifies it by bringing in more information about it.

In Indo-European languages, the modified noun phrase always precedes the relative clause. This order is reflected in the term for the modified element - *antecedent*. In fact, the order *antecedent–relative clause* is so widespread in languages that the same term is used even in languages in which the modified element comes after the relative clause, where the term *postcedent* would be more appropriate (Kordić, 1995). For example, Japanese (McCawley, 1972), Korean (Tagashira, 1972), and Basque (de Rijk, 1972) have postcedents. An antecedent can be expressed or unexpressed, as in so-called *free relatives*, e.g., English *Who has come late is hungry* ((21b) in de Rijk, 1972). The most common antecedents are nouns, as in (29), but in some languages other categories can also be relativized: for instance, adjectives can be relativized in Latin (Ehrenkranz & Hirschland, 1972), and also in Croatian, as shown in (30).

(30) Plavo, što je njegova omiljena boja, dobro mu stoji.
"Blue, which is his favourite colour, looks good on him."

A relative clause is introduced and marked by a relative word, i.e., a *relativizer*. Languages differ with respect to the types of relativizers they employ. For example, English relativizers are the pronouns *who, which*, and the complementizer *that*. Apart from relative pronouns as relativizers, relative clauses can be introduced by relative adverbs, which is the case with the Latin relative adverb of place *unde* in (31) (Ehrenkranz & Hirschland, 1972).

(31) is unde te audisse dicis
"the man whence (from whom) you say you heard it."

The antecedent of a relative clause can have different grammatical functions within a matrix clause, depending on which noun position has been relativized. According to Keenan & Comrie (1977), the hierarchy of relativizable positions is: Subject > Direct Object > Indirect Object > Oblique > Genitive > Object of Comparison (p. 66). For instance, (32) is a subject relative clause, (33) is an object relative clause, and (34) is an oblique relative clause.

(32) The tiger who scared Pi was Richard Parker.
(33) The tiger who Pi feeds every day is Richard Parker.
(34) The ship on which they travelled sank.

3.2.3.1 Cleft Sentences

Cleft sentences are a special type of relative clause. The term *cleft sentence* refers to cases where a construction divides into two parts in such a way that each of them has its own predicate (verb) (Crystal, 1985). Traditional grammar describes cleft sentences as constructions with the following structure: it + be + noun/pronoun + defining relative clause:

(35) It was Mark who chased the tiger.
(36) What he wanted to write was a book (not the article).

That usually introduces the relative clause when the object of the first clause is a proper noun, as in (37) (Thomson & Martinet, 1997).

(37) It was Anne that the tiger bit (not Mark).

3.2.3.2 Pseudo-Cleft Sentences

Pseudo-cleft sentences are a subtype of cleft sentences:

(38) The one who was invited to the party was Mark.
(39) What Mark needs is a cup of tea.

Although some languages involve cleft structuring to a very high degree (e.g., Philippine languages, see Li, 1984, p. 287), in other languages, such as Slavic, cleft and pseudo-cleft questions are almost non-existent (Comrie, 1984). While cleft and pseudo-cleft sentences are necessary means of changing focus in languages with fixed word order, such as English, Slavic languages regulate changes of focus by other means, only one of which is change in word order (Comrie, 1984). For these reasons, cleft sentences are left out from this study, which focuses on *wh*-dependencies that are more frequent in everyday communication.

3.3 *Wh*-Dependencies in Croatian

Croatian is a morphologically rich language. The morphological richness of its nominal system is reflected in the fact that this language has seven morphological cases (Nominative, Genitive, Dative, Accusative, Vocative, Instrumental and Locative), three genders (masculine, feminine, and neutral), and two numbers (singular and plural). Croatian word order is relatively free. In fact, this language tolerates any of 6 possible word orders made by combination of subject, verb and object, as in (40).

(40) Tigar lovi zebru.
tiger$_{Nom}$ chase$_{3sg.pres}$ zebra$_{Acc}$
"The tiger is chasing the zebra."

Although each example in (41)-(45) has a different word order, all of them express the same grammatical function with the same word (subject: *tiger*, object: *zebra*), and the meaning of all of them is equivalent to the meaning of (40).

(41) Zebru lovi tigar.
(42) Tigar zebru lovi.
(43) Zebru tigar lovi.
(44) Lovi zebru tigar.
(45) Lovi tigar zebru.

Smith and Mimica (1984) correctly point out that although the subject-verb-object (SVO) order in this language is very frequent, it is not clear that this is its basic word order, and propose that the language instead should be better described as a "subject-first language" (Smith & Mimica, 1984, p. 279). However, Croatian is a "pro-drop" language, which means that omission of subject in a sentence is grammatical and acceptable. Since such omissions are very common, it is also correct to describe Croatian as a (S)VO or O(S)V language, just like Italian (Bates & MacWhinney, 1987).

In examples (41)–(45), the inflectional morphology unambiguously conveys the grammatical functions of the nouns as well as the semantic relationships holding between the verb *loviti* "chase" and its arguments, i.e., the nouns *tigar* "tiger" and *zebra* "zebra". Thus: Nominative (*tigar*-ø), and Accusative (*zebr*-u) endings indicate that the grammatical functions of the nouns and thematic roles (semantic relationships) assigned to them by the verb *lovi-ti* are the following: *tigar*-subject-Agent; *zebru*-direct object-Patient.

However, Croatian grammar recognizes a few sentential elements that appear in a fixed word order. For example, clitics always appear in the second position in a sentence, although it is debatable whether the second position is the position after the first word in a sentence or after the first sentential constituent, because both are grammatically correct and acceptable (Browne, 1986; Progovac, 1996; Stjepanović, 1999). The second word clitic position in Croatian, however, breaks the constituent, as in (46), violating one of the basic principles of Universal Grammar (UG), the principle of constituent dependency (for a discussion on this, see Browne, 1986; Progovac, 1996; Stjepanović, 1999):

(46) Moj ga prijatelj poznaje.
my him_{Acc} $\text{friend}_{\text{Nom}}$ $\text{know}_{\text{3sg.pres.}}$
"My friend knows him."

(47) Moj prijatelj ga poznaje.
my $\text{friend}_{\text{Nom}}$ him_{Acc} $\text{know}_{\text{3sg.pres.}}$
"My friend knows him."

The position of clitics within a cluster is also fixed, obeying the general pattern presented in (48) (Stjepanović, 1999).

(48) li-AUX-DAT-ACC-GEN-REFL-je.

The position of clitics is also fixed within questions. For example, the clitic form of the resumptive pronoun in (49) is also in the second position in the clause.

(49) Za koga misliš da *ga* je žirafa ritnula?
for who_{Acc} $\text{think}_{\text{2.sg.pres}}$ COMP him_{Acc} $\text{Aux}_{\text{3.sg.pres}}$ $\text{giraffe}_{\text{Nom}}$ $\text{kick}_{\text{lpt.sg.f.}}$
"Who do you think that the giraffe kicked (him)?"

As a morphologically rich language with overtly marked cases and relatively free word order, which allows *wh*-dependencies of various degrees of complexity, Croatian provides an excellent opportunity to test some of the hypotheses about sentence processing found in the literature (see Chapter 5).

3.3.1 Direct *Wh*-Questions

Direct questions in Croatian do not require a specific word order, except for the *wh*-words which always appear in the initial position in single direct questions, as shown in (50), (51).

(50) *Tko* je slijedio žirafu?
Who$_{Nom}$ Aux$_{3sg.pres.}$ follow$_{lpt.sg.m.}$ giraffe$_{Acc}$
"Who followed the giraffe?"
(51) *Koju* žabu je lane liznulo?
which$_{Acc}$ frog$_{Acc}$ Aux$_{3sg.pres.}$ fawn$_{Nom}$ lick$_{lpt.sg.n.}$
"Which frog did the fawn lick?"

An exception to this rule is exemplified by interrogative sentences with an echo reading, where the *wh*-word occupies the sentence final position:

(52) Marko čita *što*?!
Mark$_{Nom}$ read$_{3sg.pres.}$ what$_{Acc}$
"Mark is reading what?!"

In multiple direct *wh*-questions, word order is again relatively free, except for the requirement that one of the *wh*-words appear in sentence-initial position, as shown in (53), (54). Syntactically, the two sentences differ only in the order of *wh*-pronouns. However, the order is semantically marked, indicating which of two referents of the *wh*-pronouns is informationally more prominent.

(53) *Tko* je koga slijedio?
who$_{Nom}$ Aux$_{3sg.pres.}$ who$_{Acc}$ follow$_{lpt.sg.m.}$
"Who followed whom?"
(54) Koga je *tko* slijedio?
who$_{Acc}$ Aux$_{3sg.pres.}$ who$_{Nom}$ follow$_{lpt.sg.m.}$
"Who was followed by whom?"

Like in English, direct questions in Croatian can have a more complex form, spreading across a single clause, as in (55).

(55) *Za koga* misliš da je lovio zebru?
for whom$_{Acc}$ think$_{2sg.pres}$ COMP Aux$_{3sg.pres}$ chase$_{lpt.sg.m.}$ zebra$_{Acc}$
"Who do you think followed the zebra?"

Croatian also forms passivized questions, as shown in (56).

(56) Tko je lovljen od tigra?
who$_{\text{Nom}}$ Aux$_{\text{3sg.pres.}}$ chase$_{\text{Pass.pt.sg.m}}$. by tiger$_{\text{Gen}}$
"Who was chased by the tiger?"

3.3.2 Embedded *Wh*-Questions

Single embedded *wh*-questions have the same structure as single direct questions, with a *wh*-word in the clause-initial position, as shown in (57) and (58).

(57) Pitam se *tko* je slijedio žirafu.
wonder$_{\text{1sg.pres.}}$ Refl who$_{\text{Nom}}$ AUX$_{\text{3sg.pres.}}$ follow$_{\text{lpt.sg.m.}}$ giraffe$_{\text{Acc}}$
"I wonder who followed the giraffe."

(58) Pitam se *koga* je tigar slijedio.
wonder$_{\text{1sg.pres.}}$ Refl who$_{\text{Acc}}$ Aux$_{\text{3sg.pres.}}$ tiger$_{\text{Nom}}$ follow$_{\text{lpt.sg.m.}}$
"I wonder who the tiger followed."

Multiple embedded *wh*-questions have relatively free word order, except that one of *wh*-words always appears in the clause-initial position. This is illustrated by the subject and object's switching of positions in (59) and (60).

(59) Pitam se *tko* je koga slijedio.
wonder$_{\text{1sg.pres.}}$ Refl who$_{\text{Nom}}$ Aux$_{\text{3sg.pres.}}$ who$_{\text{Acc}}$ follow$_{\text{lpt.sg.m.}}$
"I wonder who followed whom."

(60) Pitam se *koga* je tko slijedio.
wonder$_{\text{1sg.pres.}}$ Refl who$_{\text{Acc}}$ Aux$_{\text{3sg.pres.}}$ who$_{\text{Nom}}$ follow$_{\text{lpt.sg.m.}}$
"I wonder who followed whom."

3.3.3 Relative Clauses in Croatian

A minimal relative clause in Croatian consists of a relativizer and a verb. Croatian has declinable and indeclinable relativizers. A declinable relativizer, e.g., *koji* in (61), agrees in number and gender with its antecedent (*čovjek*), while its case depends on its grammatical function (i.e., object of the preposition *s* "with") within the relative clause.

(61) čovjek *s* *kojim* ću doći moj je brat.
man$_{\text{Nom}}$ with who$_{\text{Instr}}$ Aux$_{\text{1sg.fut.}}$arrive$_{\text{Inf}}$ my Aux$_{\text{3sg.pres.}}$ brother$_{\text{Nom}}$
"The man with whom I will arrive is my brother."

The declinable relativizers are: the nominal interrogative-relative pronouns (*tko* "who", *što* "what"), the adjectival pronouns *koji* "which", *kakav* "what kind, quality", *koliki* "how big" (size), and the possessive pronoun *čiji* "who$_{Gen}$". The indeclinable relativizers are: the indeclinable relativizer *što* "that" (not to be confused with the nominal interrogative-relative pronoun *što*), the relative adverbs *kada* "when", *gdje* "where$_{Location}$", *kako* "how" (manner), and *kuda* "where$_{Direction}$", the complementizer *da* "that", and sometimes *te* "and", "then" (Friedman, 1972; Stevanović, 1981; Browne, 1986; Kordić, 1995).

The most frequent relativizers in Croatian are *koji,* as in (61), and indeclinable *što* (Kordić, 1995). The most common indeclinable relativizer in Slavic languages in general and in Croatian in particular is a *wh*-word which very often coincides with the interrogative-relative pronoun derived from the Old-Church Slavic (OCS) *чьto* "what" (Nikolić, 1983), but its meaning as an indeclinable relativizer is "that": Russian *čto*, Ukrainian *ščo*, Byelorussian *što*, Polish *co*, Czech *co*, Slovak *čo*, Lusatian *štož,* Macedonian *što*, Bulgarian *što*, Croatian *što* (Friedman, 1972; Kordić, 1995). The indeclinable relativizer *što (što$_{IND}$)* can be used in most of the cases in which *koji* is used, as shown in (62).

(62) čovjek$_i$ *što* ću s njim$_i$ doći moj je brat.
man$_{Nom}$ that Aux$_{1sg.ft.}$ with he$_{Instr}$ arrive$_{Inf.}$ my Aux$_{3sg.pres.}$ brother$_{Nom}$
"The man that I will arrive with is my brother."

Thus, Croatian differentiates between the declinable interrogative-relative pronoun *što* (*što*$_{D}$) and the indeclinable relativizer *što* (*što*$_{IND}$), which is a conjunction. Although *što*$_{IND}$ is syntactically parallel to *koji*, it cannot be used in all the cases in which the relativizer *koji* is used. The difference between them emerges from the fact that *što*$_{IND}$, being a conjunction, cannot have an antecedent, while *koji* is a relative pronoun and thus it can have an antecedent. Yet *što*$_{IND}$ introduces a relative clause, too, expressing the syntactic function of antecedent by means of a *resumptive pronoun* - a personal pronoun co-indexed with the antecedent that *resumes* the syntactic function and meaning of the antecedent. In (62), the Instrumental form of the resumptive pronoun *he* (*njim*) is co-indexed with *čovjek*$_{Instr}$.

The resumptive pronoun and the pronominal relativizers are mutually exclusive, due to the dual nature of the pronominal relativizers, as a pronominal and a conjunction. However, in relative clauses introduced by the *što*$_{IND}$, these two functions are divided between the conjunction *što* and a pronoun itself, in this case a resumptive pronoun. There is one exception: the resumptive pronoun is never used as a subject of a relative clause, which is the "easiest" accessible role for relativizers, according to Keenan & Comrie's (1977) hierarchy. Thus, the resumptive pronoun takes over those grammatical functions that are not easily accessible to relativizers. In Croatian, the resumptive pronoun functions as a direct object whenever an antecedent refers to an animate thing, and very often when it refers to an inanimate thing. When it functions as a direct or indirect object, the resumptive pronoun takes only clitic form, as in (63), or the resulting structure is ungrammatical, as in (64); otherwise, it takes a strong pronoun form.

(63) čovjek što si *ga*$_{Acc}$ srela na zabavi
zove se Petar.
man that Aux$_{2sg.pres.}$ he$_{Acc}$ meet$_{lpt.sg.f.}$ at party$_{Loc}$
call$_{3sg.pres.}$ Refl Peter
"The man you met at the party is (called) Peter."

(64) *čovjek što si *njega*$_{Acc}$ srela na zabavi
zove se Petar.
man who Aux$_{2sg.pres.}$ he$_{Acc}$ meet$_{lpt.sg.f.}$ at party$_{Loc}$
call$_{3sg.pres}$ Refl Peter
*"The man who you met *him* at the party is (called) Peter."

It appears then that Croatian has several converging ways of conveying information on *who/which NP* that probably facilitate comprehension of the structures in which they occur. The question is to what extent these additional cues are available to aphasic population. Since *tko* and *koji* differ in several respects, it is reasonable to expect that the syntactic structures they form differ in complexity, imposing different processing demands. This book is an inquiry into how Croatian Broca's and patients with mixed aphasia comprehend *who* and *which NP* dependencies of different degrees of complexity, such as direct and embedded questions, long-distance questions with/without *za*, passivized questions, and relative clauses.

CHAPTER FOUR

SYNTAX OF *WH*-DEPENDENCIES

4.1 Chomsky's Generative Grammar

Any investigation into the nature of language, whether it involves a descriptive, analytical or computational approach, requires a theoretical framework within which linguistic structures can be defined. Most of the recent research on language in Broca's aphasia, including the study presented in this book, has adopted the theoretical framework and formalism of Chomskyan generative grammar (GG).

Following Chomsky (1957, 1965), contemporary linguists recognize two meanings of the term "grammar": first, it is a theory of language, and, second, it is a set of rules instantiated in the brain and *somehow* represented in the mind. The basic assumption that underlies generative grammar is that there is a component of the human mind/brain specialized for language[1], or, in Chomsky's terms, a *language faculty*. It is assumed that the language faculty is a uniquely human cognitive component, on one side, and that it is uniform for all human beings, on the other. In other words, human cognition has a language capacity, instantiated as Universal Grammar (UG), a potential that can be actualized throughout exposure to a particular language environment during the early age of a person's life. Depending on the language to which it is exposed, a baby will acquire a particular language. If left without any exposure to a human language, a person would not be able to actualize this language potential, and although they would still "possess" UG, they would not be able to use any particular language. Thus, UG is a set of principles inherent to language as a

[1] "We assume that the system described by UG is a real component of the mind/brain, put to use in the complex circumstances of ordinary life" (Chomsky, 1995, p. 19).

proceeds in a series of shorter steps (cycles) via intermediate Spec CP positions, leaving a trace in the original extraction site and in the intermediate Spec CP position, as in (9).

(9) $[_{CP}$ What$_i$ do you think $[_{CP}$ t_i' the frog did t_i]]?

In other words, a *wh*-word moves to the Spec CP of the clause in which it is base generated first, and then from there to the next higher Spec CP, and so on until it reaches the last Spec CP, which is the one that belongs to the matrix clause. This principle is known as the Successive Cyclic Hypothesis:

(10) Successive Cyclic Hypothesis
Long-distance *wh*-movement must proceed via all intermediate Spec CP positions.

The cyclicity of long-distance *wh*-movement is actually imposed by a deeper principle, which is known as the Subjacency Principle:

(11) Subjacency Principle
Movement must not cross more than one barrier (bounding node).

The principle states that if a *wh*-word crosses two bounding nodes (e.g., IP and NP), the resulting structure is ungrammatical. Namely, a moving element crosses a node A if A dominates its departure site, but A does not dominate its landing site. Thus, if an intermediate Spec CP is already filled, then a *wh*-word must cross two bounding nodes (barriers), and the result is an ungrammatical structure.

Wh-movement at S-structure is subject to parametric variation. Some languages have *wh*-question particles, for example Japanese (*-ka*), Mandarin (*ne*), or Korean (*ci*) (Cheng, 1997), which indicate that a clause is a question without resorting to movement. In languages without question particles, a sentence will be typed as interrogative only if a *wh*-word undergoes movement. (An exception to this rule are questions with echo reading, such as *She said what?*). In GB, this difference in forming *wh*-questions is captured by the notion of syntactic *wh*-movement. Syntactic *wh*-movement is the movement of a *wh*-word at the level of S-structure. Thus, in some languages a *wh*-word of a single question has been moved at the level of S-structure (e.g., English, Croatian), while in other languages it does not move, i.e. it stays "in situ" (e.g., Japanese, Mandarin Chinese, Korean, Hopi, Navajo, Turkish).

4.2 *Who* vs. *Which NP*

There are syntactic and processing differences between *who* and *which* types of phrases.

4.2.1 Syntactic Differences

Under certain circumstances, covert movement of *wh*-words, which takes place after S-structure, i.e., in LF, can also occur in languages with syntactic movement. In English, LF-movement occurs in multiple *wh*-constructions, where the order of extraction of *wh*-elements is constrained: the *wh*-construction that is higher up (or superior) undergoes overt movement, while the other *wh*-phrase stays in-situ: it undergoes LF movement. This condition is known as the Superiority Condition. According to this condition, a moved *wh*-element cannot cross another *wh*-element in multiple questions, as in (12).

(12) Who_i did you persuade t_i to buy what_j?

Formulated more generally, Superiority is:

(13) Superiority
"XP is superior to YP if XP and YP are in the same IP and XP c-commands YP" (Haegeman, 1991, p. 438).

This is exemplified by (14a), where the higher up or "superior" *wh*-construction *who* has been moved to Spec CP, while the lower *wh*-word, *what*, stays in situ (it undergoes LF-movement), and by (14b), which shows that the reverse order of extracting *wh*-phrases is not grammatical in English.

(14) a. Who_i t_i bought what?
b. *What_i did who buy t_i?

Pesetsky (1987) noticed that Superiority holds for *wh*-words such as *who, what*, but lexical *wh*-phrases, such as *which NP*, elude this constraint.

(15) a. Which girl_i t_i bought which book?
b. Which book_i did which girl buy t_i?

He suggested that, depending on the discourse, it is possible to distinguish between two types of *wh*-in-situ: one which moves (i.e., *which NP*), and the other which does not (i.e., *who* and *what*). Pesetsky's analysis is as follows: First, there is ambiguity in multiple questions like (16) (= (2) in Pesetsky, 1987, p. 99) due to the fact that *wh*-phrases can be "paired" differently.

(16) *Who* knows *where* we bought *what*?

In this example, both moved *wh*-phrases (*who*, and *where*) can be paired with the *wh*-in-situ (*what*). Thus, the sentence can have two interpretations: if *what* is paired with the lower *wh*-word (*where*), the narrow scope interpretation will follow and an answer to the question (16) will have the form as presented in (17a). If, on the other hand, *what* is paired with the higher *wh*-word (*who*), the wide scope interpretation will follow and an answer will have the form as in (17b):

(17) a. *John* knows where we bought what (the book in Amsterdam, the record in Groningen, etc.)

b. *John* knows where we bought the *book* (in Amsterdam); *Mary* knows where we bought the *record* (in Groningen); etc. (= (3) Pesetsky, 1987, p. 99).

Second, Pesetsky presents two different accounts of the ambiguities occurring in (16): Baker's (1970), and Chomsky's (1975) approach. Baker (1970) represents the scope of all *wh*-phrases by co-indexing them with the Q morpheme in the Comp of interrogative clause (Comp corresponds to CP in later terminology), and the scope of the phrase is determined by co-indexing with either the lower or the higher Q. Narrow-scope representation is shown in (18a), where *what* is coindexed with the lower Q, along with *where*. The wide-scope representation is shown in (18b), where *what* is coindexed with the higher Q, with *who*.

(18) a. $[[_{Comp}$ Q_j $who_j]$ e_j knows $[[_{Comp}$ $Q_{i,k}$ $where_k]$ we bought $what_i$ $e_k]]$
b. $[[_{Comp}$ $Q_{i,j}$ $who_j]$ e_j knows $[[_{Comp}$ Q_k $where_k]$ we bought $what_i$ $e_k]]$

For Chomsky (1976), all *wh*-words are in Comp at the LF level, and the scope of the *wh*-phrase depends on the Comp in which the phrase appears, as shown in (19) (Pesetsky 1987). In (19a), *what* appears in the lower clause with *where*; in (19b) it appears in the higher clause with *who*.

(19) a. [[$_{\text{Comp}}$ who$_j$] e_j knows [[$_{\text{Comp}}$ what$_i$ where$_k$] we bought e_i e_k]]
b. [[$_{\text{Comp}}$ what$_i$ who$_j$] e_j knows [[$_{\text{Comp}}$ where$_k$] we bought e_i e_k]]

Based on these analyses, Pesetsky proposes that some *wh*-in-situ phrases, such as *which NP*, behave as proposed by Baker, i.e. "without movement but with unselective binding, like indefinites", while *wh*-in-situ phrases such as *who* and *what* behave as proposed by Chomsky – "with movement at the level of LF, like real quantifiers" (for example, *who* and *what*) (Pesetsky, 1987, p. 103).

Structurally, the two types of *wh*-phrases have different positions within their phrases: *which* is a specifier inside its NP, while *who* and *what* are heads of the phrase, as shown in (20a, b).

(20) a. b.

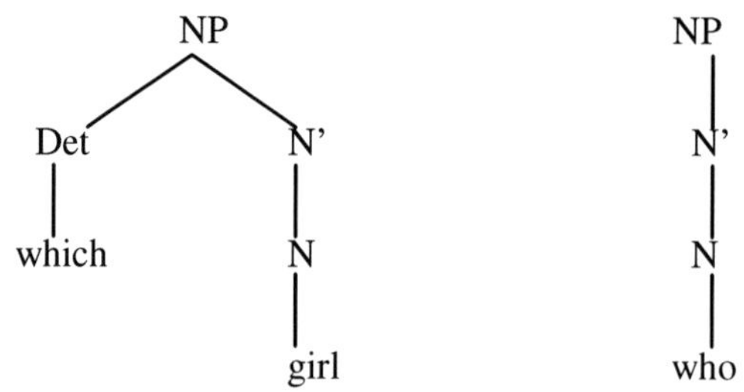

However,

> … the crucial difference between a *which*-phrase and the *normal* occurrence of *who* or *what* is found in discourse. ... Roughly, *which*-phrases are *discourse-linked (D-linked)*, whereas *who* and *what* are normally not D-linked. When a speaker asks a question like *Which book did you read*?, the range of felicitous answers is limited by a set of books both speaker and hearer have in mind. If the hearer is ignorant of the context assumed by the speaker, a *which*-question sounds odd (Pesetsky, 1987, p. 107-108).

In other words, the scope of non-D-linked *wh*-phrases in situ is determined by movement at LF. Since D-linked *wh*-phrases in situ do not move, overtly or covertly, their scope is assigned by a different mechanism: co-indexation (Pesetsky, 1987).

The differences between the two types of questions are summarized in the table below (Avrutin, 1999; Balogh & Grodzinsky, 1996; Cinque, 1990; Hickok & Avrutin, 1996; Pesetsky, 1987; Hagiwara, 1993).

Table 4-1: *Who* vs. *Which NP* questions

Who/What Qs	*Which NP Qs*
Chomsky-style analysis	Baker-style analysis
Behave as quantifiers	Behave as indefinites
Non-D-linked	D-linked
Form government chains	Form binding chains
Non-referential	Referential
Move at LF when in-situ	Do not move at LF when in-situ
Obey syntactic constraints	Obey syntactic & discourse constraints
Head movement	Phrasal movement

4.2.2 Processing Differences

Pesetsky's discourse-related distinction between *who, what* and *which NP* questions suggests that the two types of questions should differ in terms of processing as well. The processing difference would reflect the fact that in addition to syntactic constraints, D-linked questions obey discourse related constraints, such as shared presuppositions on the discourse and other elements of common ground of conversation.

Psycholinguistic evidence confirms that the two types of questions differ in terms of processing. As an example, in a reading study with neurologically intact native speakers of Italian, De Vincenzi (1996) found a difference in processing of subject and object *who* vs. *which NP* questions: *who* questions were better comprehended than *which* questions, and subject questions were better comprehended than object questions. Frazier and Clifton (2002) argue that, unlike non-D-linked phrases, D-linked phrases are immediately represented in a discourse representation in addition to a syntactic representation, demonstrating for instance that readers preferred D-linked to non-D-linked phrases as pronoun antecedents.

Avrutin (2000), building on insights from Hickok and Avrutin (1996), claims that the integration of the syntactic and discourse knowledge may be computationally more demanding than processing of non-D-linked phrases. Since this approach takes into consideration both the structural constraints and the processing demands of *wh*-questions, it is considered as a possible explanation of English-speaking Broca's aphasics' chance performance on D-linked object questions (see Sections 4.3.3.1 and 4.3.3.2).

4.3 The Syntactic Comprehension Deficit in Broca's Aphasia

Evidence from Broca's aphasia has shown that focal brain injury can selectively impair a person's ability to perform syntactic computations. However, it is not clear how much Broca's area contributes to which type of syntactic computations and what additional brain areas support syntax. In the following sections I present the general pattern of the comprehension deficit in Broca's aphasia as well as the *who/which NP* pattern, and explanations proposed on them.

4.3.1. The General Pattern

The finding that Broca's aphasics can correctly judge grammaticality of a sentence without being able to understand its meaning (Linebarager et al., 1983) has had impact on the development of the idea that agrammatism is a partial loss of syntax. Namely, some researchers proposed that these patients fail to represent only specific elements of syntactic structure (Grodzinsky, 1986, 1990; Mauner et al., 1993; Hickok et al., 1993). Emerging from this view, a specific pattern of comprehension deficit in Broca's aphasia was discerned that was based on the concept of canonicity.

Canonicity involves the matching of two hierarchies: a thematic roles hierarchy (Agent > Patient/Beneficiary > Theme > Source/ Goal) and a grammatical function hierarchy (subject > direct object > indirect object). In a canonical sentence structure the two hierarchies match in the sense that the highest NP in one hierarchy is associated with the highest NP in the other, the next NPs in both hierarchies match, and so on. In an SVO language such as English, the two hierarchies match in an active sentence, such as (23).

(23) The boy kissed the girl.

The order of thematic roles (Agent *the boy* – Patient *the girl*) matches the order of grammatical functions (subject *the boy* – object *the girl*). In non-canonical sentence structures, such as passive sentences, object relative clauses, or object cleft sentences, there is a mismatch between thematic hierarchy and grammatical function hierarchy, as illustrated in (24).

(24) The girl was kissed by the boy.

Here *the girl* is the grammatical subject, but (since it is the logical object) is assigned the thematic role of Patient[4]. The role of Agent is assigned to the indirect object, *the* boy, which altogether produces a mismatch between the thematic roles order (Patient–Agent) and the order of grammatical functions (subject–indirect object).

It has been claimed that Broca's aphasic patients comprehend canonical sentence structures (25a-c) at a level greater than chance, while they perform at chance level on tasks involving comprehension of non-canonical sentence structures (26a-c) (Caramazza & Zurif, 1976; Hickok et al., 1993; Mauner et al., 1993; Grodzinsky et al., 1999; Inglis, 1999; Grodzinsky, 2000b; Piñango, 2000a).

(25)
(a) The girl kissed the boy.
(b) The girl that kissed the boy is tall.
(c) It was the girl that kissed the boy.

(26)
(a)The boy was kissed by the girl.
(b) The boy that the girl kissed is shy.
(c) It was the boy that the girl kissed.

However, the claim that Broca's aphasics perform above chance level in comprehension of canonical sentences and at chance level in comprehension of noncanonical sentences has been questioned in light of the debate on single case studies vs. group studies in research on language disorders (Berndt, Mitchum & Haendiges, 1996; Grodzinsky et al., 1999; Berndt & Caramazza, 1999; Zurif & Piñango, 1990; Caramazza, Capitani, Rey & Berndt, 2001; Drai & Grodzinsky, 1999; Drai, Grodzinsky & Zurif, 2001; Zurif, 2001; Caplan, 2001). The debate centres on whether the pattern of comprehension deficit in agrammatic Broca's aphasia that has been repeatedly reported in group studies actually holds, given the randomness in performance of agrammatic Broca's patients reported in single case studies (Druks & Marshall, 1995). Thus, it has implications for the methodology employed in the two types of studies.

Although the debate focuses on whether to confirm or reject the proposed general pattern as a whole, it is mostly based on reports on

---

[4] In order to avoid terminological confusion due to a variety of labels for this role (e.g., object, objective, goal, theme, patient and so on), as discussed by Blake (1994), in this book I use the term Patient and differentiate between the roles *Patient* and *Theme*.

Broca's aphasics' comprehension of semantically reversible passive sentences. In a review of 15 studies on the comprehension deficit in Broca's aphasia published between 1980 and 1993, Berndt et al. (1996) found that only 36% of the patients reported in those studies understood active sentences above chance, and passive sentences at chance level, while the remaining 64% showed above chance performance on both conditions (30%) or chance performance on both conditions (34%). Thus, according to their analysis, only one third of Broca's patients in these studies actually confirmed the pattern (with regard to active-passive sentences), which renders the canonical-noncanonical pattern of comprehension deficit in agrammatic Broca's aphasics implausible. Not only does the reported pattern not hold, but also the randomness in patients' performance suggests that group studies may not be reliable, and perhaps should be dismissed in favour of single-case studies (Berndt et al., 1996; Caramazza et al., 2001).

However, a review by Grodzinsky and his colleagues (Grodzinsky et al., 1999) of the relevant literature published between 1980 and 1996 showed that "Broca's patients, as a group" confirm the canonical-noncanonical pattern of the comprehension deficit, thus supporting group studies of language disorders (Zurif & Piñango, 1999). They noticed that only some of the agrammatic patients in Berndt et al.'s (1996) review were actually diagnosed as Broca's aphasics by some standardized test, suggesting that the pattern may hold only for agrammatism in Broca's aphasia, and not for "agrammatism on its own".

Nevertheless, there are other reports on a Broca's agrammatic comprehension deficit that do not fit the pattern. Hickok et al. (1993) found that, contrary to the pattern, the comprehension of a matrix clause in center-embedded relatives with a predicate-adjective relation, such as (27), was impaired in Broca's aphasics. This sentence is difficult to process because in addition to determining who is chasing whom, patients have to determine who is fat.

(27) <u>The cat</u> that chased the mouse <u>is fat.</u>

Also, the empirical evidence has shown that comprehension of passives in agrammatic Broca's aphasics is not always impaired. For instance, Druks and Marshall's (1995) patient B.M. comprehended passive sentences above chance, while his comprehension of active sentences was at chance. Inglis (1999) observed that patient C.V. comprehended off-line passives, whereas this patients's on-line comprehension of passives was impaired, which indicates a processing rather than the structural impairment.

Lukatela et al. (1995) showed that 4 out of 7 Serbo-Croatian speaking Broca's agrammatic aphasics comprehended object relative sentences above chance.

4.3.2 *Who/Which NP* Pattern

Another puzzling finding comes from the research on Broca's aphasics' comprehension of *wh*-questions involving *who* and *which NP* types of questions. Hickok and Avrutin (1996) found that Broca's aphasics' performance on direct questions was better than chance on tasks including both subject and object *who* questions, while their comprehension of *which NP* questions was asymmetric, with better than chance performance on tasks involving subject *which NP* questions and chance performance on tasks with object *which NP* questions. That is, Broca's aphasics' comprehension of *which NP* questions was consistent with the prediction of the general pattern: better comprehension of subject relatives, subject clefts and therefore subject *which NP* questions than object relatives, object clefts, and therefore object *which NP* questions. However, Hickok and Avrutin's patients' comprehension of *who* questions was not correctly predicted by this general pattern, because their comprehension of object *who* questions was above chance.

Tait et al. (1995) and Thompson et al. (1999) tried to replicate the *who* vs. *which NP* comprehension pattern in Broca's aphasics reported by Hickok and Avrutin (1996). Their respective findings are that only 2 out of 4, and 1 in 4 patients followed the reported pattern. Salis and Edwards (2008) did not find this pattern in the comprehension of *wh*-structures in 5 English-speaking Broca's aphasics they tested. Neuhaus and Penke (2008) found that 3 out of 9 German-speaking Broca's aphasics followed the *who/which NP* pattern. French-speaking Broca's aphasics also exhibit difficulty in comprehension (as well as in production) of object *wh*-questions; for them, *wh*-questions formed by *wh*-movement are more difficult than *wh*-in-situ questions (Van der Meulen, Bastiaanse & Rooryck, 2005). Thus, even though there may be only a subset of agrammatic Broca's aphasics who exhibit the *who/which NP* comprehension asymmetry, the pattern is interesting and needs to be explained. I first review the explanations proposed for the general pattern, since they are the basis of the *who/which* NP explanations.

4.3.3 Explanations Proposed

4.3.3.1 General Pattern

Grodzinsky (1986, 1990) proposed that the selective loss and sparing in the comprehension deficit pattern in Broca's agrammatics is a consequence of their inability to establish traces at the level of S-structure, which further results in their failure to assign thematic roles to the moved elements. Without the thematic roles, they cannot interpret meanings of the sentential constituents or infer the meaning of a sentence in general. Grodzinsky's proposal on trace deletion, known as the Trace Deletion Hypothesis (TDH), is theoretically anchored in GB and based on the concept of syntactic displacement. Recall that the movement of a constituent (e.g., NP) leaves a trace behind in the position of the moved element. In GB, a trace is an abstract, phonologically empty element, a "space-holder" with a twofold function: (1) to receive a thematic role from a verb; and (2) to assign the received thematic role to the moved element with which it is co-indexed.

As they are unable to access thematic roles of the moved elements to interpret a sentence, Broca's aphasics resort to a cognitive strategy consisting of assigning the role of Agent to the first available NP in the sentence (Grodzinsky, 1990, 1995). For example, passive sentences such as *The boy was kissed by the girl* will be interpreted as *the boy* = Agent, *the girl* = Patient. In other words, the role of Agent is assigned to the first available NP in the sentence by default, which in the case of active sentences results in an adequate interpretation, but in passive sentences does not, leading to chance performance. Thus, although Broca's agrammatic patients fail to assign thematic roles properly, they can actually comprehend canonical sentences, because these are syntactically already ordered in a way that coincides with the Agent-first strategy.

(28) Trace Deletion Hypothesis (Grodzinsky, 1986, 1990, 1995):
(a) Traces of moved arguments are deleted in the Broca's agrammatic representations.
(b) An NP lacking a thematic role due to trace deletion is assigned a thematic role by a linear default strategy (e.g., the Agent role is assigned to the clause initial NPs).

Thus, the TDH predicts that the interaction between impaired syntactic representations (containing no argument traces) and the default strategy

(Agent first) results in Broca's agrammatic aphasics' comprehension deficit in noncanonical sentences.

Both assumptions on which the hypothesis is built are to some extent problematic. The basic prediction of the TDH, that Broca's aphasic patients cannot represent traces at S-structure because they cannot deal with syntactic displacement, seems to be too general (Hickok et al., 1993; Mauner et al., 1993). Although all three types of non-canonical sentences (passives, object-relatives and object-clefts) are formed by movement from object position, the Agent-first strategy will only correctly predict that Broca's aphasics have difficulty comprehending passives, since assigning the role of Agent to the first NP in object-relatives, (29), and object-clefts, (30), will actually produce the correct response. Broca's aphasics, however, do not perform above chance on these structures: they do not know who chased whom in (29) and they think that the cat chased the dog in (30).

(29) The cat that the dog chased is brown.
(30) It was the cat that the dog chased.

Thus, the TDH does not make correct predictions about object-relatives and object-clefts, and cannot explain the asymmetry in Broca's aphasics' impaired comprehension of object relative clauses and object-clefts and their relatively preserved comprehension of subject relative clauses and subject-clefts (Piñango, 2000b).

Also, it has been claimed that the default interpretive strategy postulated by the TDH is an ad hoc, extralinguistic mechanism without the capacity to determine where in the course of processing, and why, comprehension of moved object relatives breaks down (Hickok & Avrutin, 1993; Mauner et al., 1993; Piñango, 2000b). It has been criticized for being designed to explain the deficit for the specific canonical word order found in English, and for not being "independently motivated", i.e., it cannot be proved that the same strategy is used by children or by other populations who show difficulty with the same type of constructions (Crain, Ni & Shankweiler, 2001; Friederici & Gorrell, 1998). Thus, not only is the TDH unable to explain the general pattern, but being methodologically tied to aphasic comprehension, it furthermore lacks the potential to expand into a processing theory.

Hickok et al. (1993) and Mauner et al. (1993) have suggested that TDH can be improved by adopting the VP-Internal Subject Hypothesis. According to this hypothesis, grammatical subjects in English are base generated within the VP; they move out of the VP to the Spec IP, creating a chain which consists of the moved element and its trace.

(31) [$_{IP}$ The tiger$_i$ [$_{VP}$ t$_i$ chased the zebra]].

Hickok et al. (1993) and Mauner et al. (1993) suggest that by adopting this hypothesis the TDH can completely dispense with the default strategy. As it stands, the only difference between the subject-gap and object-gap sentences that the TDH can make is related to the position from which these elements are extracted (i.e., subject-gap sentences are formed by movement from a subject position, and object-gap sentences are formed by movement from object position).

Thus, the TDH adopts the idea that there is only one movement - from object position, and hence one type of chains. However, adopting the VP-Internal Subject Hypothesis means that, in addition to the movement from object position, there is also a movement from subject position. This further means that there are two types of chains, and that grammatical subjects also receive their thematic roles via a trace.

This approach also postulates a thematic assignment representation (TAR), predicting above chance comprehension of sentences with only one NP that can be assigned an unsatisfied thematic role. In cases with two or more NPs that can be assigned an unsatisfied thematic role, comprehension results in chance performance. The new proposal, that Broca's agrammatic aphasics cannot link antecedents and traces in the syntactic analysis, is known as the Revised Trace-Deletion Hypothesis (RTDH).

4.3.3.2 Proposals on *Who/Which NP* Asymmetry

Hickok and Avrutin (1996) were the first to report the *who/which NP* pattern in Broca's aphasics' comprehension: good comprehension of both subject and object *who* questions, as well as subject *which NP* questions, but poor comprehension of object *which NP* questions. Their explanation of the pattern focused on the nature of *who/which NP* phrases, and in particular on the specific features of *which NP* phrases: their property of being D-linked, and their ability to form binding chains. Since their patients did not show asymmetry in comprehension of subject vs. object *who* questions, Hickok and Avrutin concluded that only binding chains are disrupted in Broca's aphasia. For example, in (32), Broca's aphasics would have a problem comprehending only (32d):

(32) a. Who t chased the zebra? - Non-D-linked subject *wh*-question
b. Who did the tiger chase t? - Non-D-linked object *wh*-question
c. [Which tiger] t chased the zebra? - D-linked subject *wh*-question
d. [Which zebra] did the tiger chase t? - D-linked object *wh*-question

Since the initial traces in (32b) and (32d) occupy the same positions in the structure, the position of the trace itself cannot explain why the former is comprehended above chance, while the latter is comprehended at the chance level (Grodzinsky, 2000b). However, the type of chains the traces of *who* and *which NP* enter into with their respective antecedents, according to Hickok & Avrutin (1996), can explain the asymmetric pattern: binding chains (*which NP*) are unbounded and can be established over long dependencies, which makes them computationally more demanding than the government chains (*who, what*), which are only locally constrained, and thus easier to process (see Section 4.2.1).

Several elements of Hickok & Avrutin's study have been criticized in the literature: the disruption of binding chains hypothesis (a) leaves unanswered why (32b) is comprehended above chance, (b) does not generalize to Broca's aphasics' deficit in comprehension of passives (Balogh & Grodzinsky, 2000), and (c) referentiality was tested in an act-out task, which may not provide appropriate informational context (Thompson et al., 1999).

Another explanation of the *who/which NP* asymmetry in Broca's aphasia is proposed by Grodzinsky (1995) in a revision of his original TDH.

(33) Trace Based Account (TBA) (Grodzinsky, 1995)
a. Trace deletion: Traces in theta-positions are deleted from agrammatic representations.
b. R(eferential)-strategy: Assign a referential NP a role by its linear position if it has no thematic role (p. 44).

The default R-strategy applies only to referential NPs, which, in the case of our two types of *wh*-questions, means only to *which NP* questions. On the other side, *who* is non-referential and as such is exempted from the R-strategy. This is a subtle, but important change in traced-based approach, because it allows the TBA to capture the asymmetry in the comprehension pattern of subject-object extracted *wh*-questions. Thus, according to the TBA, in examples like (32d) the R-strategy assigns the role of agent to the first referential NP - *which zebra*. Since the verb *chase* also assigns the role of agent to *the tiger*, the sentence contains two agents resulting in the performance at the chance level. This is not the case with the non-D-linked (32b) questions: since *who* is non referential, it does not obey the R-strategy; so *the tiger* is properly assigned the agent role, and comprehension is above chance.

However, Tait et al. (1995) and Thompson et al. (1999) suggest a different explanation for the *who/which NP* asymmetry. In an attempt to replicate Hickok & Avrutin's results, they found that only two of four agrammatic subjects showed the *who* versus *which NP* asymmetry (Tait et al., 1995). Their explanation is based on the semantic representation of the questions they tested. For example, questions (34-36) show above chance performance on both subject and object extractions and have the representation (37), which involves a single computation:

(34) Who kicked the elephant?
(35) What kicked the elephant?
(36) Which one kicked the elephant?
(37) FOR WHICH X, kick-elephant (X)

Questions with *which NP* expression such as (38) have one more predication relation, as shown in (39), which poses difficulty to agrammatic aphasics:

(38) Which giraffe kicked the elephant?
(39) FOR WHICH X, giraffe (X) AND kick-elephant (X)

However, Hickok and Avrutin do not consider object extracted *which NP* questions semantically more difficult. Since *which* NP questions refer to an already known set of propositions from which one needs to be selected, and thus is smaller than the set of propositions for *who*, *what* questions, the former are easier to answer than the latter (Hickok & Avrutin, 1996). In addition to trying to replicate the results of Hickok & Avrutin's study, Thompson et al. (1999) also tested TBA, which predicts Broca's aphasics above chance comprehension of passivized subject *who*, chance comprehension of passivized subject and object *which NP* questions, and below chance comprehension of passivized object *who* questions. They found that "none of the subjects" performed as predicted by TBA (Thompson et al., 1999, p. 180).

Thompson et al. (1999) briefly mention a possible approach based on Chomsky's (1995) Minimalist Program, a further development to GB theory. The Minimalist Program distinguishes between *who* and *which NP* questions in terms of movement, with the former involving head movement, and the latter, phrasal movement. Although they related the distinction to Hagiwara's (1995) evidence that head movement is intact in Broca's agrammatic aphasia, it is not clear how exactly adopting the distinction would explain the data on the *who/which NP* pattern collected so far.

It appears, then, that all attempts to explain comprehension of *wh*-dependencies in Broca's aphasics within a syntactic framework fall short of their goal in some way. In Chapter 5, I examine approaches to processing of *wh*-dependencies.

CHAPTER FIVE

PROCESSING COST OF GAP FILLING

Although the structural syntactocentric conception of language architecture is prominent, it is not the only theoretical framework within which one could explore language deficits. An alternative approach is to analyse language as a dynamic interplay among cognitive components, and determine in what ways and to what extent each of them contributes to language processing.

Sentence comprehension is a complex process that requires fine-tuning and synchronizing of several processes: auditory/visual word recognition, lexical and morphological processes, syntactic analysis or parsing, conceptual interpretation, and referential processes (Kempen, 1998). Being so complex, it relies heavily on the memory systems, among which a memory subsystem that temporarily stores and processes information in serving higher mental processes is especially important (Jonides & Smith, 1997; Stowe et al., 2002)[1].

5.1 Working Memory

In the broadest sense, memory is the storage and retrieval of information. The term *memory* is twofold, referring at the same time to the knowledge that is stored in the brain, and the processes by which this knowledge is acquired and stored (Tranel & Damasio, 1995). Over the last 40 years, psychological research on memory has provided considerable evidence for the existence of two basic memory systems: the long-term memory (LTM) and short-term memory (STM) systems. The LTM system is a complex of subsystems that are functionally specialized for different tasks[2]. Behavioral studies, neuropsychological evidence and evidence

---

[1] Parts of this chapter appeared in my paper *Is Syntactic Working Memory Language-Specific*? published in *Psihologija* (2010), *43(1),* 71-87.

[2] Despite the lack of consensus on the exact structure of the LTM system, there is evidence on different types of LT memories: e.g., knowledge about the world

from neuroimaging studies all converge in suggesting that short-term memory also fractionates into functionally different subsystems.

The term *working memory* (WM) has been in use since the work of Miller, Galanter and Pribram in the 1960s and was adopted in the Baddeley and Hitch's three-component model in the 1970s (Baddeley, 2003). It was intended to emphasize the difference between a unitary model of STM as a passive storage of information and the dynamics of the three-component model, which combined the idea of the multicomponential nature of STM with the view that this limited-capacity system not only stores, but also processes information, facilitating higher cognitive functions, such as reasoning, learning, and comprehension (Baddeley, 2003). In this functional architecture of memory, WM is functionally open to any type of information that needs to be stored for a very brief period of time. Due to its limited capacity and fast processing, WM deals with fragile information, which however can be quickly accessed and updated (Jonides & Smith, 1997).

Baddeley and Hitch's concept of WM consists of three components: the phonological loop, the visuo-spatial sketchpadd and the central executive. The first component stores and processes verbal information, the second visual information, while the third is a controlling attentional component, which controls the first two components (Baddeley, 1990, 2000). More recently, the episodic buffer has been added to the model; its function is to store and bind information into integrated episodes (Baddeley, 2003).

The phonological or articulatory loop stores and processes verbal information. It takes in auditory or written material, transforms it into a phonological code and registers it in the phonological store. Since the phonological store holds memory traces for approximately 1.5-2 seconds, another process within the phonological loop takes over: the subvocal rehearsal. Namely, after a memory trace fades away, it can be refreshed "by a process of reading off the trace into the articulatory control process which then feeds it back into the store, the process underlying the subvocal rehearsal" (Baddeley, 1990, p. 72).

Based on the assumption that the phonological record of the whole sentence is necessary for accurate assignment of thematic roles to the nouns in a sentence, early research on the role of the phonological loop in sentence comprehension assigned it a critical role. However, the early

---

(semantic memory), memories of events from a person's life (episodic memory) (Tulving, 1972), memory supporting various skills, such as riding a bike or applying the rules of grammar (procedural memory), etc. For fractionation of LTM, see Tulving (1972) and Tranel and Damasio (1995).

psycholinguistic findings showed that incoming verbal material is being analysed as a sentence is perceived (Frazier & Fodor, 1978). Further research showed that sentence repetition requires more than phonological storage, and that, as a matter of fact, semantic representation of a sentence is even more important in tasks such as repetition (Martin & Romani, 1994). Caplan and his colleagues propose that although the phonological loop does not play a role in the first pass analysis of a sentence, it is important in the second pass when, confronted with several possible interpretations of a sentence, a listener needs to decide which one to choose (Caplan & Waters, 1999). In line with this view is other researchers' claim that the phonological loop does not play an important role in sentence comprehension, although it can contribute to it by ensuring verbatim repetition of information (Martin & Romani, 1994; Chein, Ravizza & Fiez, 2003). Although the phonological loop has been investigated much more than other components of WM (Baddeley, 2003), its role in sentence comprehension remains controversial (Van der Linden & Poncelet, 1998).

Comprehension of complex syntax requires that contents of intermediate representations be temporarily stored so that different processes can operate on them. These intermediate syntactic representations contain abstract elements (such as traces) necessary for establishing syntactic hierarchical and dependency relations. Sentence comprehension requires that syntactic and semantic processes be applied to sequences of sentential elements so that hierarchy among the elements and dependency relations within the sentence are established, and further representations deduced.

If linguistic theory is correct in postulating a trace, a phonologically empty and silent element that serves as a space-holder for syntactically displaced elements within an intermediate representation, as psycholinguistic evidence also suggests, then the question is: Can the phonological loop, a WM component consisting of phonological storage and subvocal rehearsal, recognize a trace and leave a space for it within a sequence? More importantly, can it store and process information on the chain that the moved constituent and its trace form, and the type of relationship they enter? If not, then some other component of WM must be engaged in processing of syntactic dependencies.

A possible candidate supporting this type of processing is the central executive system. The central executive, which is the least developed component of the model, is a processor oblivious to the informational domain. It is supposed to be a set of processes that control computations being performed on the contents of WM. However, the concept of central executive is still vague (Baddeley, 2003). Since comprehension of complex syntax crucially depends on WM, a more specific model of a syntactically relevant WM component that enables temporary storage and processing of syntactic structures is preferred to the model in which a concept as wide as the central executive is responsible for syntactic processes.

Caplan and Waters (1999) proposed a finer distinction within the WM system: it contains subsystems that are engaged in different types of verbal tasks. For instance, discerning a message from a linguistic signal represents interpretive processing (e.g., word recognition, parsing, assignment of thematic roles, etc.) and is supported by a WM subsystem different from the one that supports so-called post-interpretive processing, which operates when meaning is used to accomplish other tasks, such as reasoning, planning, learning, and so on. Caplan et al. (2000) have shown that syntactically complex sentences were associated with increased rCBF in Broca's area; however, this increase was not due to phonological rehearsal, but rather due to activation of WM resources supporting syntax.

Theories of sentence processing emphasize the importance of "structuring a sequence of words syntactically and semantically" for its interpretation (Gibson, 1998, p. 2), i.e., building a grammatical structure according to the rules of grammar, from which intended meaning of a sentence can be inferred (Kempen, 1998). Theories of sentence processing differ from other fields of language processing (single word reading, spoken word production, etc.) in being completely divorced from neuropsychological research (Martin & Miller, 2002). The same criticism holds for theories on sentence comprehension in aphasia – they are disconnected from theories of normal sentence comprehension (Zurif et al., 1993; Friederici & Gorrell, 1998). This is puzzling, given that very often researchers from both areas share the same linguistic framework and formalism (e.g., generative grammar), and are interested in similar topics (e.g., syntactic displacement). Comprehension of *wh*-dependencies in agrammatic aphasia is an excellent opportunity to test theories that have the potential to bridge the gap between theories of sentence processing in intact and damaged brains.

5.2 Working Memory and Syntactic Computation

One such a theory is the Syntactic Prediction Locality Theory (henceforth SPLT) proposed by Gibson (1998). The SPLT focuses on the relationship between the parser (sentence processing mechanism) and the available computational resources provided by WM. The idea that comprehension can be limited due to limitations of WM resources is not new, and has been confirmed in normal (Daneman & Carpenter, 1980; Just & Carpenter, 1992; Vos et al., 2001) and aphasic populations (Miyake, Carpenter & Just, 1994, 1995; Caplan & Waters, 1995, 1996; Haarmann, Just & Carpenter, 1997) as well as in children (Gaulin & Campbell, 1994). However, researchers do not agree on the nature of WM resources. Some of them, inspired by the work of Just & Carpenter (1992), argue for a single-pool concept of WM resources, while others gravitate towards a multi-component concept of WM, where different components control different aspects of sentence processing (e.g., semantic WM, syntactic WM, etc.) (Martin & Romani, 1994; Martin, 1995; Caplan & Waters, 1999).

Even when they do not agree on the theoretical framework within which they conduct their empirical work, researchers on sentence processing usually agree that certain syntactic relations (e.g., dependencies) and operations (e.g., syntactic displacement in structures with subject- vs. object-extractions) are computationally more demanding than other syntactic relations and operations. For example, a syntactic operation such as movement of a sentential constituent requires the human sentence processor to hold the displaced element in WM until it encounters its trace/subcategorizer (Felser et al., 2003).

In SVO (Subject-Verb-Object) languages, such as English, comprehending a declarative sentence with canonical SVO word order, as in (1), poses less computational demand than comprehension of an interrogative sentence, as in (2):

(1) Mary likes *White Teeth*.
(2) *Which book* does Mary like t?

Since (1) has a canonical SVO word order (subject-verb-object), a direct object (*White Teeth*) immediately follows the verb *like*. However, (2), being a question with a fronted *wh*-object, has a noncanonical structure; it thus places a greater computational demand on the parser because readers/ hearers cannot assign a grammatical interpretations to the fronted *wh*-expression until they establish a syntactic dependency relation between *which book* and its trace, nor can they assign a thematic role to *which book* until they encounter the verb *like*. Thus, the processing cost depends on the distance between the dislocated element (*which book*), also called *filler* (i.e., the antecedent), and its subcategorizing verb, as well as on the distance between the filler and a *gap* (i.e., the trace left behind and marked by *t* in the example above). It is also possible that, in addition to the processing load created by these two relationships, the nature of material that intervenes between the filler and its gap/subcategorizing verb contributes to the processing load.

The two relationships, filler–gap and filler–subcategorizer, are critical in sentence processing. The process of forming an association between a filler and a gap is called gap filling (Pickering & Barry, 1991). The nature of the relationship between the filler and its subcategorizer (verb or preposition) has provoked a debate in the literature (e.g., Pickering & Barry, 1991; Gibson & Hickok, 1993; Gorrell, 1993; Pickering, 1993; Hawkins, 1999; Fiebach et al., 2002), resulting in two models of sentence processing. The representatives of the Empty Category Model of sentence processing claim that the association between the moved constituent and its subcategorizer crucially depends on the extraction site (Gibson & Hickok, 1993; Gorrell, 1993), while the advocates of the Direct Association Hypothesis (DAH) argue against empty categories in human sentence processing, claiming that the moved constituent is directly associated with the subcategorizer (Pickering & Barry, 1991; Pickering, 1993).

Thus, processing of complex syntax involves a significant amount of computational load, imposing great demands on WM. Experimental work using Event Related Brain Potentials (ERP) has shown that a specific effect – an early left anterior negativity (LAN) with a latency of about 300 to 500 msec was elicited when filler-gap constructions were processed (Kluender & Kutas, 1993). This finding was interpreted as an indication that the moved element was identified and held in memory until the processor reached this element's original position in the sentence. The effect was reported for object relative clauses (King & Kutas, 1995) and for other types of noncanonical sentences (Rösler et al., 1998). Since the moved element has to be held in memory until the parser reaches its original position in the sentence, it was hypothesized that the LAN effect reflected syntactic WM processes that support on-line storage and manipulation of information related to the syntactic movement.

Gibson (1998) has developed the idea that the processing cost consists of two separate components: a memory cost and an integration cost. The memory cost component determines the amount of computational resources needed to store "a partial sentential input", while the integration cost component determines how much of the computational resources needs "to be spent on integrating new words into the structures built thus far" (Gibson, 1998, p. 8). In other words, the memory cost depends on the number of syntactic predictions about the lexical categories that have to be held in WM, while the integration cost depends on the number of new discourse referents. The key constraint on both memory cost and integration cost is locality: the syntactic predictions held in memory for a longer period of time and integrations over longer distances are more expensive. Thus, the parser critically depends on WM processes for establishing the filler-gap relation. In examples such as (2), temporary storage of a moved constituent, its retrieval from WM, and its integration with the subcategorizing verb - all contribute to the processing cost (Felser et al., 2003; Fiebach et al., 2001, 2002).

Wh-dependencies are a typical example of syntactic structures that require storage of unintegrated information and its on-line manipulation in establishing the filler-gap and filler-subcatogorizer relationships. Fiebach et al. (2002) conducted ERP experiments on the comprehension of embedded *wh*-questions in German. As mentioned earlier, unlike English, which is an SVO language, German is a verb-final language (SOV). In English, a subcategorizing verb is followed by a direct object gap, and the thematic role of a moved element cannot be established before a dependency relation between the moved element and its subcategorizing verb is established. This makes it difficult to determine in English whether the processing cost depends more on the relation between the subcategorizer and the moved element, or on the link between the moved element and its trace.

This is not the case with SOV languages like German where the subcategorizing verb occupies the sentence final position. According to the Active Filler Strategy (Frazier & Clifton, 1989), the parser will establish syntactic dependencies as early as possible, which in the case of SOV languages means that the parser is able to establish the dependency relation between the filler and its gap before the verb is encountered. Since German marks grammatical functions of NPs by overt case endings, it is possible that grammatical functions are determined before the subcategorizing verb has been processed (Felser et al., 2003). (However, thematic roles can be assigned to the filler only after the subcategorizing verb has been encountered.) This makes it possible to explore the dissociation between the memory cost (which depends on the relationship between the moved constituent and its trace) and the integration cost (which depends on the relationship between the moved element and its subcategorizer) in German, but not in English.

Indeed, Fiebach et al. (2002) found that case-unambiguous embedded German object *wh*-questions with a longer distance between the antecedent and its trace, as in (4), elicited a specific ERP effect as a consequence of greater computational load in processing: a sustained left anterior negativity (LAN) appearing around 400 msec after the onset of the first prepositional phrase (PP).

(3) Thomas fragt sich, *wer* am Dienstag nachmittag nach dem Unfall den Doktor verständigt hat.
Thomas asks himself who_{Nom} on Tuesday afternoon after the accident the_{Acc} doctor called has.
"Thomas is wondering who called the doctor on Tuesday afternoon after the accident."
(4) Thomas fragt sich, *wen* am Dienstag nachmittag nach dem Unfall der Doktor verständigt hat.
Thomas asks himself, who_{Acc} on Tuesday afternoon after the accident the_{Nom} doctor called has.
"Thomas is wondering who the doctor called on Tuesday afternoon after the accident."

Since the same type of object questions but with a shorter distance, subject questions, as in (3), and gap-free control sentences did not elicit a similar response, they conclude that the LAN is the effect of processing a very specific type of syntactic construction: it reflects the memory cost of keeping the moved *wh*-constituent over a longer distance in WM. Thus, the syntactic WM cost depends on the distance between the antecedent and its trace, and additionally it is influenced by individual WM capacity.

Another processing step - integration of the moved element into a phrase structure representation - elicited another ERP component. Namely, a positive ERP component between 300-600 msec was found at the second NP [*Doktor*] in both types of object questions, short and long, but not in subject questions (Fiebach et al., 2002). These findings indicate different processing costs in embedded short vs. long subject vs. object German questions. Since LAN and the positive-going ERP effect are two different ERP components, they indicate that two different WM mechanisms are involved in processing object questions: syntactic memory cost and syntactic integration cost, respectively (Fiebach et al., 2002). Their findings also run against the DAH, which would predict a greater processing cost on the verb, instead of at the NP *Doktor* in (4).

Felser et al. (2003) took a step further in exploring the two types of processing costs by trying to resolve whether the memory cost is determined linearly or hierarchically, i.e., whether the distance depends on the number of words that intervene between the antecedent and the trace, or on the hierarchical organization of the phrase structure. In order to determine if the distance is linear or structure-dependent, Felser et al. (2003) compared the ERPs elicited by the processing of three types of structures: *wh*-object movement, long-object topicalization, and raising and object topicalization, plus a control structure consisting of short object topicalization. Their results support the claim that the LAN reflects the memory cost, and a positivity around 600 msec (P600) reflects the integration cost. Additionally, they found that the memory cost, unlike the integration cost, was not influenced by the type of dependency (e.g., *wh*-movement vs. topicalization) that holds between the filler and the gap. However, it depended on the syntactic complexity of the elements intervening between the filler and the gap.

5.3 Case Inflection and Syntactic WM

In addition to syntax (the length of distance between the filler and the gap and the type of intervening material), languages with rich morphology employ features of morphological subsystems in processing. For instance, case endings indicate grammatical roles and are associated with thematic roles. The memory cost, i.e., the processing cost of the filler-gap relationship, would be smaller in such languages than in languages that rely exclusively on syntax, such as English.

Consider the relationship between the dislocated element and its trace in (4) above. The ERP evidence suggests that this relationship can be established before the verb is encountered. Namely, the LAN effect occurred at the dislocated element, *wen*, and lasted until the NP *Doktor* was reached. At this point in the sentence, i.e., immediately before the trace, the sustained negativity "was almost not observable any longer" (Fiebach et al., 2002, p. 268). This suggests that, although *wen* is unambiguously case marked for the object position within the VP, it is held in WM until the parser encounters the NP *Doktor,* and not the verb. Based on this evidence, Fiebach et al. claim that overt case marking can trigger some syntactic processes which otherwise require information available from the verb. Felser et al. (2003) reached the same conclusion. However, the LAN component in their study was not sustained, but rather indicated that the moved element was reactivated at the gap position. Regardless, the data indicate that it is reasonable to assume that the difference in position at which a subcategorizing verb projects a gap in English (post-verb position) and in German (pre-verb position) imposes differences in processing of the filler-gap relationship in these languages.

Analogously, given the structural differences between English and Croatian, we may expect differences in processing of the same relationship in these two languages. Like German, Croatian employs case endings to indicate grammatical roles, but a gap typically, although not necessarily, appears after the verb, like in English (i.e., if unmarked informationally).

Although the gap in (4) also follows the verb as in (2), the Croatian counterpart of the sentence in (2) does not depend that much on syntax:

(5) *Koju knjigu* Meri voli t?

Namely, *koju knjigu*, being marked for case, gender and number, contains more information than *which book*. Since the Accusative case, marked by the suffix *–u*, unambiguously indicates that the filler must be linked with the object position of the VP, the parser can assign the grammatical function of object to the NP in the sentence initial position as soon as it encounters the suffix in *koj-u*. In other words, relying on the morphological information contained in the inflectional ending *-u*, the parser can immediately determine grammatical function of the dislocated element and predicts its gap, without resorting to the syntactic information conveyed by the distance between the moved element and its trace.

Since the processing cost depends on the distance between the moved element and its trace, it can be increased by either syntactic complexity of the intervening material (e.g., the intervening material has additional levels of linguistic structure) or by the linear increase of the distance (e.g., by multiple insertions of the same-level phrases). This means that sentences involving two types of movement (e.g., passivized questions in Experiment 4) or those in which an element moves cyclically across the whole sentence (over clauses, as in long-distance questions in Experiment 2) pose more processing load than sentences with one type of within-clause movement (such as direct questions in Experiment 1).

Also, a greater processing cost is expected in structures such as (4) above, where it is manipulated not by increase in hierarchical complexity, but by linear extension, i.e., adding of multiple PPs (as in Experiment 3). Due to its relatively free word order, Croatian allows and tolerates a structural equivalent of (4), as shown in (6), although the sentence with the auxiliary *je* moved to the position immediately after *koga* shown in (7) contains a word order more typical for Croatian. The position of the auxiliary *je*, however, does not affect the filler-gap relationship either in (6) or in (7).

(6) Tomas se pita koga u utorak popodne nakon nezgode doktor zvao je.
Thomas asks himself who$_{\text{Acc}}$ on Tuesday afternoon after the accident doctor$_{\text{Nom}}$ AUX$_{\text{3sg.pres.}}$ call$_{\text{lpt.sg.m.}}$.
"Thomas is wondering who the doctor called on Tuesday afternoon after the accident."

(7) Tomas se pita koga *je* u utorak popodne nakon nezgode doktor zvao.
Thomas asks himself who$_{Acc}$ AUX$_{3sg.pres.}$ on Tuesday afternoon after the accident doctor $_{Nom}$ call$_{lpt.sg.m.}$
"Thomas is wondering who the doctor called on Tuesday afternoon after the accident.

Since the processing cost also depends on morphological information conveyed by the inflectional endings, it seems plausible that processing of structures such as (6) and (7) is easier in grammars with unambiguously case marked NPs. We hypothesize that, based on the case-marking of a clause initial filler (*-ga* in *koga* in (6) and (7)), the parser predicts a grammatical role of the moved *wh*-word (a direct object), and thereby a position of the gap within a VP, predicting also the filler's thematic role (Patient). In other words, the parser constructs a preliminary syntactic structure, which is checked when the parser encounters a verb.

The question which is still open is: What exactly is held in WM? Clifton and Frazier (1989) proposed that WM holds either the filler itself or some of its features. For Gibson (1998), it is the parser's predictions on constituents of a minimal grammatical clause. One could also claim that the parser employs features of the filler in constructing a partial syntactic representation of a minimal grammatical clause.

For example, although *tko* and *koji NP* share some features, such as [+ *wh*] and [+ case], they can be distinguished with regard to the following features:

(8) [+/- D-linked], [+/- gender], [+/-number].

Thus, the features [+wh], [+ D-linked], [+Accusative], [+ masculine], [+ singular] make up:
(a) lexically: *kojeg NP*,
(b) grammatically: direct object,
(c) thematically: Patient (or Theme).

If [+wh], [+ D-linked], [+ Nominative], [+ masculine], [+singular], then:
(a) lexically: *koji NP*,
(b) grammatically: subject, and
(c) thematically: one of the following roles, for instance:
(i) Agent: *Koji dječak pjeva?* "Which boy is singing?"
(ii) Beneficiary: *Koji sin je naslijedio kuću?* "Which son has inherited the house?"

(iii) Source: *Koji roditelj mu je dao auto?* "Which parent gave him a car?"
(iv) Theme: *Koji roman imaš na umu?* "Which novel is on your mind?"
(v) Patient: *Koji susjed je orobljen?* "Which neighbour has been mugged?"

The combination of features [+wh], [- D-linked], [+Acc], [-gender], [- number] is realized as follows:
(a) lexically: *tko*,
(b) grammatically: direct object,
(c) thematically: Patient (or Theme).

If [+wh], [- D-linked], [+Nom], [-gender], [- number], then:
(a) lexically: *tko*,
(b) grammatically: subject,
(c) thematically: one of the following roles, among others:
(i) Agent: *Tko pjeva?* "Who is singing?"
(ii) Beneficiary: *Tko je naslijedio kuću?* "Who has inherited the house?"
(iii) Source: *Tko mu dade auto?* "Who gave him a car?"
(iv) Theme: *Tko ti je na umu?* "Who is on your mind?"
(v) Patient: *Tko je orobljen?* "Who has been mugged?"

Since words are sequences of morphemes, it is possible that bound morphemes whose repetition is required by agreement are processed faster and with smaller amount of resources than those that need to be matched without such repetition. For instance, the same ending *-a* on the noun and adjectives strung in a phrase such as *bratova nova bijela košulja* "brother's new white shirt" indicates that each of these four words have the same case (Nominative), gender (feminine), and number (singular). Similarly, the suffix *-a* in *Koja košulja?* "which shirt" carries a repetition of information on the case, gender and number in the *wh*-pronoun and noun.

5.4 Syntactic WM and Broca's Aphasia

Gibson's (1998) distinction between the memory cost and the integration cost seems a more promising starting point than the general idea that limited WM influences sentence processing, when addressing the question of how different cognitive systems interact to enable complex tasks imposed by language. Some researchers are reluctant to rely on proposals that explain sentence processing in terms of WM, given that a "fully specified" model of WM has not been proposed yet (Stowe et al., 2002). Others more readily accept ideas such as Gibson's, developing models of syntactic processing around them. Fiebach et al. (2001, 2002) are building a specific theory of sentence processing based on the concept of syntactic working memory (SWM), which intends not only to link different cognitive systems, but also to ground thus construed functional architecture in neuroanatomy. Fiebach et al. (2001) argue that:

> [...] there exists a separate cognitive or neural resource that supports syntactic working memory processes necessary for the temporary maintenance of syntactic information for the parser. In the context of *wh*-movement, such a memory component is necessary for establishing filler-gap dependencies (p. 321),

and that:

> syntactic working memory, rather than syntactic processing per se, is supported by Broca's area (p. 321).

As discussed in Chapter 2, there is growing evidence suggesting that a specific part of Broca's area subserves syntactic operations that are computationally more demanding, such as those involved in syntactic movement. Evidence also shows that this area does not support only syntactic computations in language processing; rather it supports a variety of tasks. It is possible that the area that was once claimed to subserve only computations required for comprehension of sentential dependencies actually has a more general purpose, supporting the sequential processing of structurally dependent elements. In this view, the concept of syntactic WM would need to be reconsidered and possibly extended from syntax of language to syntactic computations in other cognitive domains.

If syntactic knowledge is preserved in Broca's aphasics, and yet there is a breakdown in establishing some, presumably more demanding types of sentential structures (e.g., long distance object *wh*-questions or extended embedded questions), then it seems reasonable to link the breakdown in syntactic comprehension with the role of WM in processing. One of the research questions in this study is whether a greater distance, in terms of number of elements involved between the moved element and its trace, affects comprehension of *wh*-dependencies in Croatian aphasics in any significant way. In particular, Experiment 3 is an adaptation of Fiebach et al.'s (2002) experiment for testing Croatian aphasic patients.

If the hypothesis that Broca's area is the locus of syntactic movement (Grodzinsky, 2000b) or that it subserves SWM processes (Fiebach et al., 2001) holds, then one would expect to find differences in comprehension of *wh*-dependencies in aphasic patients with a lesion in this area compared to normal controls. Additionally, since Broca's and other aphasics have limited processing resources, structures that impose a greater processing load should be difficult for them to comprehend, even if they do not have a lesion exactly in Broca's area.

CHAPTER SIX

PRESENT STUDY

6.1 Research Questions

The present study investigates whether the pattern of asymmetric comprehension of *who* and *which NP* dependencies displayed by English-speaking Broca's aphasics (Hickok & Avrutin, 1996) exists in Croatian-speaking Broca's aphasics. Although several different structural proposals have been presented, the asymmetric pattern reported by Hickok and Avrutin, set within the context of a general pattern of syntactic deficits in this population, still has not been explained (see Chapters 4 and 8). Contributing evidence on comprehension of *wh*-dependencies in aphasic speakers of a structurally different language, such as Croatian, may shed new light on the issue.

There are three possible outcomes of the search for the asymmetry in comprehension of subject vs. object *who/which NP* dependencies in Croatian Broca's aphasics:

A. There is no asymmetry in comprehension of subject vs. object *who/which NP* structures in Croatian Broca's aphasics.
B. There is asymmetry in comprehension of subject vs. object *who/which NP* dependencies in Croatian Broca's aphasics and it matches the asymmetric pattern found in English-speaking Broca's aphasics.
C. There is asymmetry, but it does not match the asymmetric pattern reported for the English-speaking Broca's aphasics.

Given the structural differences between English and Croatian, and the results of previous studies on Croatian Broca's aphasics' comprehension abilities, this study tests the hypothesis that a possible subject-object asymmetry in comprehension of *who* and *which NP*-dependencies in Croatian Broca's aphasics does not match the asymmetric pattern reported for English Broca's aphasics. In order to test the hypothesis, and in light of the theoretical background presented in Chapters 2-5, the present study seeks answers to 3 questions:

1) If the subject-object asymmetry exists in *who/which NP* dependencies in Croatian Broca's aphasics, is it determined hierarchically or linearly?

If it is determined hierarchically, then greater syntactic complexity would have more impact on Croatian aphasics' comprehension of *wh*-dependencies. If it is determined linearly, then greater distance, in terms of number of elements involved between the moved element and its trace, would affect their comprehension in a significant way. Experiments 1, 2 and 4 test aphasics' comprehension of *wh*-dependencies in structures of different degrees of complexity: direct, embedded, long-distance and passivized questions formed by *tko* "who" and *koji NP* "which NP", and relative clauses introduced by *koji* "which". Experiment 3 tests the impact of a greater distance on comprehension of *wh*-dependencies in Croatian aphasics.

Moving towards more general issues, I explore the following two questions:

2) Which component(s) of the underlying cognitive mechanisms implicated in the processing of *wh*-dependencies need(s) to be deficient for emergence of the particular comprehension pattern of subject-object asymmetry, or *who-which NP* asymmetry, if they exist?
3) Can we draw any reliable conclusions about the relationship between these mechanisms and the lesion site in each patient, and can we make any further generalizations regarding the cognitive mechanisms involved in processing of complex syntax?

6.2 Methods

6.2.1 Testing Paradigms in Previous Studies on Syntactic Comprehension Deficit in Broca's Aphasia

Studies on the syntactic comprehension deficit in Broca's aphasia often rely on a single paradigm, and sometimes combine two or more off-line behavioral paradigms, such as sentence-picture matching, act-out, and grammaticality-judgement paradigms (e.g., Linebarger et al., 1983; Grodzinsky, 1995; Hickok et al., 1993; Hickok & Avrutin, 1996; Thompson et al., 1999). While research based on off-line paradigms has contributed valuable insights on Broca's aphasics' comprehension abilities, research on comprehension deficits in aphasia using on-line behavioural paradigms also contributed important observations. For instance, a cross-modal lexical priming (CMLP) technique was used to test the hypothesis that slow lexical access causes the syntactic comprehension disturbances in Broca's aphasia (Prather et al., 1991; Zurif et al., 1993; Swinney et al., 1996). Only recently have on-line methods, such as Event-Related Brain Potentials (ERP) and neuroimaging techniques like Positron Emission Tomography (PET) and functional Magnetic Resonance Imaging (fMRI), been applied in studying syntactic comprehension deficits in Broca's aphasics (Swaab et al., 1997; Karbe et al., 1998; Marchand, D'Arcy & Connolly, 2002). While these methods have changed our understanding of when and where in the brain certain language processes take place (Kljajevic, 2011a), they are not readily available to a wider research community. In addition to general challenges associated with each of these methods (e.g., PET requires use of a radioactive tracer, which allows only a limited number of stimuli during one session; fMRI machines produce a great amount of noise and, due to their construction may trigger claustrophobic experience in patients), there are also specific challenges associated with using these methods with post-stroke patients (e.g., conducting ERP experiments requires extra time for electrode positioning, which may exceed the amount of time a patient is able to participate in experiments). As a consequence, behavioral methods, such as grammaticality judgments, sentence-picture matching, and act-out paradigm, still dominate research on post-stroke aphasia.

A paradigm based on grammaticality-judgment has been used in the assessment of a specific aspect of sentence structure—its grammaticality (Linebarger et al., 1983). Studies based on this paradigm have shown that English-speaking Broca's agrammatic patients, in spite of their comprehension deficits, can correctly judge the grammaticality of sentences (Linebarger et al., 1983). Like English aphasics, Serbo-Croatian aphasics have shown relatively good performance on grammaticality judgments of subject and object relative clauses (Lukatela, 1989; Milekić, 1993).

One explanation of this finding is that judging a grammatical structure is computationally less demanding than comprehension (Zurif et al., 1993). Earlier research on "split-brain" patients showed that the right hemisphere could perform grammaticality judgments, but it could not support syntactic comprehension. This finding motivated another view, according to which judging grammaticality, being supported by the right hemisphere, is spared in right-handed Broca's aphasics, whereas syntactic comprehension, which is supported by the left hemisphere, is impaired in these patients.

In a sentence-picture matching task, a subject is required to judge if the meaning of a sentence is correctly represented by one of several pictures. For example, in the case where semantically reversible sentences are tested, a patient is required to select from a pair of pictures the one that best represents the meaning of an auditorily presented sentence (Berndt et al., 1996; Inglis, 1999). Since semantic reversibility is crucial in assessing comprehension, a set of distributed pictures usually contains a picture that represents correct assignment of thematic roles to sentence nouns, and a distracter picture showing a reversal of thematic roles assigned to the nouns in a sentence, resulting in an incorrect meaning of the sentence. One problem with this paradigm is that it imposes unnecessary computational load (Hickok et al., 1993): in addition to sentence parsing, this type of task also requires that two or more pictures be parsed and compared. This is typically not present in sentence comprehension in the everyday use of language. Another problem with this type of testing is that sentences are presented out of context: creating a context necessary to interpret such sentences also represents an unnecessary computational burden (Hickok et al., 1993).

Another often-used paradigm in testing Broca's comprehension deficit is the act-out paradigm. In an act-out task, a subject "acts out" an auditorily presented sentence with toys (animals or dolls) (Caplan & Futer, 1986; Hickok & Avrutin, 1996; Inglis, 1999). In other words, a subject is required to manipulate a toy to demonstrate, or enact the action of a verb in a spoken sentence. However, this type of task reduces the discourse from a set of potentially infinite number of possibilities to a limited number of alternatives manageable within the testing paradigm. It also imposes certain non-linguistic cognitive demands (Inglis, 1999), such as memory, and non-cognitive ones. A non-cognitive factor, but equally important as the cognitive ones, pertains to the fact that aphasia following left hemisphere damage is often associated with restricted motor agility of the right arm in a patient, which may dramatically reduce the outcome of the act-out task. The same restriction may also affect the outcome of on-line comprehension testing methods that require fast and accurate movements as a response, making them inappropriate for comprehension studies in these patients (Müller et al., 1997).

A version of an act-out task that can be applied in testing aphasic subjects with reduced motor agility is the truth-value judgment task (Hickok et al., 1993). In this version of the act-out paradigm, a scenario is acted out by the experimenter, after which a sentence is read. The subject is required to decide whether the sentence correctly represents the situation acted out or not, and to say or point to a sign indicating either "true" or "false". In this case, the subject attends to a sentence rather than a picture, and accepts or rejects a sentence, instead of a correct or incorrect picture, which is the case with the sentence-picture matching task. This simplifies the sequence of cognitive and non-cognitive subtasks a patient needs to perform in order to successfully complete the task. Since a patient watches the experimenter acting-out the task, it takes less time for a sentence to be acted out. Not only is the amount of time that a patient needs to store a sentence in WM shorter, but his/her motor activities are reduced to simple pointing, leaving him/her a chance to fully concentrate on the sentence, instead of performing a motor task. Thus, this version of the act-out task is less demanding cognitively (less memory, less attention, no interference of cognitive and non-cognitive requirements) and non-cognitively (smaller motor effort). Since this version of act-out task avoids the factors that would be confounded with syntactic processing in the previous version of the task as well as in picture-matching task, it has been used in three experiments in this study.

6.2.2 Testing Paradigms in the Present Study

In order to investigate comprehension of *wh*-dependencies in Croatian Broca's aphasics, in this study I use the "pointing" version of the act-out paradigm in Experiments 1, 2, and 4. In addition, a test of auditory sentence comprehension and the role of WM in it, based on the verification paradigm, is employed in Experiment 3. The verification paradigm consists of the following: a sentence is auditorily presented to a participant, after which a probe assertion is read. Each probe assertion is a short active sentence whose meaning is contained in the sentence being tested, only manipulated with regard to truth/falsity by switching the nouns in subject and object positions. The participant is required to decide whether the probe assertion is true or false with respect to the target sentence, and to say (or point to a sign indicating) "True" or "False". For example, the sentence *Peter knows which patient called the doctor on Tuesday afternoon* could have either of the following probe assertions: *The doctor called the patient* or *The patient called the doctor.* Thus, the task requires comparing the sentence representation and the representation of a probe assertion, and deciding whether the assertion is contained in the sentence or not (i.e., whether it is true or false).

6.2.3 Type of Study

The four experiments in this study[1] test for comprehension of *who/which NP* dependencies in eight native Croatian aphasic patients and three control subjects. The result is a series of case studies on aphasia caused by stroke. Except for a broad generalization concerning their language deficit, the patients who participated in the study differ in type of aphasia, exact site of lesion, age, and post-onset time. This information is summarized in Table 6-1, and details on each case are provided in Chapter 7.

Several reasons contributed to choosing the case study approach. First, focusing on a single case or on several individual cases, instead of studying a group, solves the problem of inter-individual variability within a syndrome. Generalizations on each individual case are then made with regard to a loosely defined syndrome, as discussed in Chapter 2, allowing a greater degree of "grey areas" between the types of aphasia. This reflects clinical reality much better than theoretical classifications, which force cases with mixed characteristics into clear-cut categories, i.e. syndromes.

Second, the major batteries of tests for assessment of aphasia that have been translated into Croatian still lacked standardization and appropriate adaptation of the material to the Croatian language at the time of testing. Lack of reliable test batteries made it difficult to categorize Croatian aphasics into existing types of aphasia. Here we rely on the reports of speech pathologists and medical documentation that were made available for the purposes of this research, aiming at a more precise characterization that can follow only from a detailed description of the nature of language deficit in each patient.

The study was approved by the Ethics Committee at Carleton University, Ottawa, and the local hospitals' authorities in Zagreb, Croatia. It was conducted in accord with the Declaration of Helsinki.

6.2.4 Aphasic Participants Profile

Only post-stroke aphasic patients participated in this study, and all but one had had an ischemic stroke. The decision to choose participants with the same etiology was motivated by the fact that different etiologies may display different features of language deficit.

---

[1] Part of the data presented here have been published in Kljajevic & Murasugi (2010) and Kljajevic (2010).

All the aphasic subjects were outpatients, with at least 6 months post-onset time, which is the minimum time necessary to achieve language stability (Ferro & Madureira, 2002). There was no limit with regard to how much longer than 6 months they had been recovering. The participants were chosen among high-functioning aphasics, who were able to pay attention to a task for sufficient time. Those who could not complete the *Introductory session* or the trial questions in the subsequent session, either because they did not understand instructions on how to realize the tasks, or because their attention span would not allow them to complete even short blocks of testing, such as those in trials, did not qualify as potential participants. Aphasic patients with other conditions, such as blindness, deafness, or dementia, were not eligible for the study either. One aphasic patient who could not engage into a "pretense" atmosphere required by the enactment task with the toy animals was excluded from further testing[2]. All participants had normal or corrected to normal vision and none had reported hearing problems. They all signed a written consent before the testing began.

The eight aphasic patients were clinically diagnosed with the following:

- anomic aphasia (S.T.),
- Broca's aphasia (M.N., A.D, and P.J.),
- mixed nonfluent aphasia (T.P., B.R. and J.Z.), and
- mixed fluent aphasia (K.S.).

Only S.T. and A.D. did not display characteristics of agrammatic speech; the remaining six aphasics were agrammatic to differing extents.

The eight Croatian aphasic stroke patients consisted of five male and three female subjects. At the time of testing, they were between 51 and 78 years old. Their education varied between 11 and 16 years. The native language of each participant was Croatian; however, before their illness, all of them were fluent in one or more other languages. The post-onset time in each case met the general criterion of at least 6 months as the minimal time necessary for achievement of language stability. They varied from 6 months to 2 and half years, with the exception of one case where the post-onset time was around 7 years. Lesion site in each case was on the left side, with the exception of one patient (A.D.) in whom it was bilateral. An ischemic stroke caused aphasia in all of the cases, except in patient B.R., who had an intracerebral hemorrhage. All of the subjects

[2] Tłokiński (1995) reports on similar reactions in illiterate people and children.

were right-handed, but patient M.N. was ambidextrous. This information is summarized in Table 6-1.

Table 6-1: Aphasic Participants Profile

Case	Age	Sex	Edu	Post-onset	Lesion site	Aphasia
ST	57	F	12	9 m	LPCA	anomia
MN	51	M	16	28 m	LMCA	Broca's
AD	78	F	12	12 m	L+ RICA	Broca's
PJ	60	F	16	31 m	LMCA	Broca's
TP	54	M	16	20 m	LICA	mixed nonfluent
JZ	74	M	16	7 y, 2 m	LMCA	mixed nonfluent
BR	59	M	14	15 m	LBG	mixed nonfluent
KS	65	M	11	6 m	LMCA	mixed fluent

Abbreviations used in Table 6-1:
Edu. = years of formal education.
Lesion site:
L&RICA-Left & Right Internal Carotid Artery; LPCA-Left Posterior Cerebral Artery; LBG-Left Basal Ganglia; LMCA-Left Middle Cerebral Artery; LICA-Left Internal Carotid Artery.

The patients were recruited through speech pathologists at the Neurological Clinic at *Bolnica Sestre Milosrdnice* and at the Policlinic *SUVAG* in Zagreb.

6.3 Evaluative Measures

The Raven's Coloured Progressive Matrices Test (RCPM), the Digit Span (backward), and a set of tests from the Boston Diagnostic Aphasia Evaluation (BDAE) were used to evaluate participants' non-verbal intelligence, short-term memory span, and their general syntactic comprehension abilities.

6.3.1 The Raven's Coloured Progressive Matrices Test (RCPM)

RCPM (Raven, 1976) is a standardized, non-verbal measure of intelligence, highly correlated with verbal IQ. The reason for administering an intelligence test was to determine whether language difficulties in aphasic patients represent selective language impairment. This is usually the case when there are discrepancies between results of intelligence tests and aphasia tests. However, Kertesz and McCabe (1975) found that Broca's, transcortical motor, conduction, and anomic aphasics performed better on the RCPM than Wernicke's, transcortical sensory and global aphasics. Their finding indicates that non-verbal intelligence is not totally spared in aphasic population. The reason for choosing the RCPM in the present study was its non-verbal nature, which makes task performance less dependent on verbal information. The test consists of three parts, with each part containing 12 different visual patterns. Each visual pattern has one section missing, which needs to be completed from a selection of six similar patterns (only one of them fits the overall pattern). The subject receives one point for each correct pattern selected, with the maximum score of 36 points. The experimenter marks each score on a sheet of paper provided with the test. The test takes approximately 15 minutes to complete.

6.3.2 Digit Span (Backward)

The Digit Span task (Backward) from the Wechsler Adult Intelligence Scale-Revised (WAIS-R) (Wechsler, 1981) was administered for measuring STM span employed in general tasks. The Digit Span is used in the present study as a general test of STM span. It involves repeating, in reverse order, a string of numbers verbally presented by the experimenter. The number of digits in the string is increased by one with each turn, starting from two and going up to eight. A simple manipulation of reversing elements in a string requires good storage capacity. The test is relevant for the present study because in order to establish syntactic dependencies within a sentence, the parser requires certain memory span. It takes 5-10 minutes to complete the test.

6.3.3 Boston Diagnostic Aphasia Evaluation (BDAE)

The aphasic patients who participated in this study underwent a neurological exam, CT scanning, and assessments by speech pathologists. They had not been evaluated in a comprehensive examination modelled after tests such as the BDAE or Western Aphasia Battery. Instead, a speech pathologist followed a series of assessing procedures that resulted in a descriptive characterization of a patient's language deficit. Each patient was assessed by a speech pathologist at three different levels. The first assessment was usually brief, based on a short, screening test similar to *Norsk Grunntest for Afasi*, "Norwegian Basic Aphasia Assessment", (Reinvang, 1985), and it was administered after the patient had been admitted to a hospital. The scores of this test, however, usually are not kept, as the only purpose of the test is to facilitate descriptive reporting of a patient. The second assessment is thorough. It is performed at a rehabilitation hospital, where aphasic patients stay for three weeks. During that time the patient is engaged in an intensive, individual therapy designed specifically for his/her language profile. Since most aphasic patients recover their language performance during the first few weeks after stroke, the primary goal of this intensive, individual therapy is to enhance the potential for recovery. As a consequence, the results of the third assessment performed by a speech pathologist with whom a patient will work after rehabilitation may differ from the first two.

Aphasia, just like a lesion causing it, evolves. Vignolo (1988) argued that a post-stroke lesion is typically relatively stable about after 21 days post-onset and that it takes about 21-60 days post-onset to reduce diaschisis and compensation. Similarly, Alexander et al. (1990) pointed out that analysis of only early CT scans "may involve considerable risk of a missing lesion still evolving or overestimating as lesion what is actually just transient edema" (p. 360). To remedy this situation, they recommended that CT scans be taken again two or more months after stroke. Ojemann (1991) has also emphasized the "temporal instability" of early post-stroke findings and the fact that "language deficits may change over time after the patient suffers from a particular brain lesion" (p. 2282).

Since the scores of initial testing were not available, parts of the BDAE related to syntactic comprehension were administered to the aphasic participants in this study. The purpose of this was not to try to classify aphasics into syndromes. Even when fully tested, aphasic patients are classified into different aphasia types with a degree of uncertainty: Goodglass and Kaplan (1983) point out that in some centers only about 30% of aphasic cases can be unambiguously classified into syndrome types, although in other centers this can be 80% of cases. Spreen & Risser (2003), probably applying the concept of aphasic syndromes in a stricter way, claim that only 20% to 30% of aphasic speakers can be reliably classified. Some aphasic patients cannot be classified at all (Willmes & Poeck, 1993). In those patients who are classified, aphasia often evolves, requiring re-classification. As an example, Willmes and Poeck (1993) observed that out of five patients with large lesions who were initially classified as global aphasics four evolved to Broca's and one to anomic aphasia. Thus, the purpose of administering portions of the BDAE to Croatian-speaking aphasic patients was rather to determine if there was a correlation between their performance on the BDAE comprehension tasks and the comprehension tasks employed in this study. Croatian translation and adaptation of the following BDAE Auditory Comprehension subtests were administered: *Word discrimination*, *Body-part identification*, *Commands*, and *Complex ideational material*.

6.3.4 Other Evaluative Tests of Comprehension

Some of the *Supplementary Language Tests* accompanying the BDAE were also used, such as *Passive subject-object discrimination, Contrast: indicative-interrogative,* and *Asking questions* (*Yes-No questions* and *Wh-questions*) (Goodglass & Kaplan, 1983, pp. 51-57). The reason for administering the *Supplementary Language Tests* was to obtain further information on aphasic patients' abilities to comprehend complex syntax relevant for the present study, because it has been shown that patients with mixed non-fluent aphasia have more pronounced comprehension deficit than Broca's aphasic patients. For instance, the tested structures included examples like "*If I tell you 'The lion was killed by the tiger', which animal is dead?*" (passive subject-object discrimination), "*How would you ask me if it is raining?*" (Yes-No question), and "*How would you ask me what the weather is outside?*" (*wh*-question). For each correct answer on these tests participants received 1 point, with the maximum score of 5 for passive subject-object discrimination and asking questions, and 10 points for the indicative vs. interrogative repetition task.

Finally, four more types of sentences were administered as an evaluative test. Since Experiment 3 contains probe assertions with *netko* "someone" and *neki NP*, a set of 20 sentences was administered within the *Introductory session* specifically to test for comprehension of *netko* and *neki NP*. In addition, declarative passive sentences with and without the preposition *by* were tested as a pre-test to the experimental testing of passive questions in Experiment 4. Examples of the pre-test stimuli are given in Table 6-2.

Table 6-2: Examples of pre-test comprehension stimuli

Sentence type	Examples of pre-test stimuli
Declarative active *netko*	Netko je preskočio lava. "Somebody jumped over the lion."
Declarative *neki NP* passive-*by*	Neki tigar je liznut. "A tiger was licked."
Declarative passive-no-*by*	Zebra je ritnuta. "The zebra was kicked."
Declarative passive-*by*	Zebra je ritnuta od žirafe. "The zebra was kicked by the giraffe."

6.4 Experimental Measures

6.4.1 Goals

In order to test the hypothesis presented in Section 6.1, four experiments were specifically designed to answer the following questions:

General Question 1:
Does the subject-object asymmetry exist in Croatian Broca's aphasics' comprehension of *who* and *which NP* dependencies?

General Question 2:
Do Croatian Broca's aphasics comprehend better *who* or *which NP* dependencies?

All experiments include the following 4 variables, where *tko* is "who" and *koji NP* is "which NP": subject *tko*, object *tko*, subject *koji NP*, and object *koji NP* (Table 6.3).

Table 6-3: Variables

	Who	*Which*
Subject	tko	koj-i, a, e (NP)
Object	koga	ko(je)-ga, u, e (NP)

The experiments differ in the syntactic constructions within which these variables appear. The questions each experiment was designed to test with regard to General Question 1 are as follows[3]:

1) Experiment 1: Does the subject-object asymmetry exist in direct and embedded *who* and *which NP* questions, and in relative clauses introduced by *which*? Namely, this experiment tests aphasics' comprehension of direct and embedded subject-object *tko/koji* NP questions, as well as comprehension of subject-object relative clauses introduced by the relativizer *koji.*
2) Experiment 2: If the subject-object asymmetry exists in *wh*-dependencies, is it determined hierarchically? The experiment tests aphasics' comprehension of long-distance subject-object *who/which*

[3] See Section 3.3 for a description of *wh*-dependencies in Croatian and Tables 6-4.1 to 6-4.4 for examples of experimental stimuli.

NP questions. The experiment contains two variants of *who* and *which NP* long-distance questions: *tko/koji NP* questions without the *za* and *tko/koji NP* questions with the preposition *za.*

3) Experiment 3: If the subject-object asymmetry exists in *wh*-dependencies, is it determined linearly? Experiment 3 attempts to answer this question by testing whether greater distance, in terms of number of elements involved between the moved element and its trace, affects comprehension of *wh*-dependencies in any significant way. More specifically, Experiment 3 tests for aphasics' comprehension of embedded subject-object *who/which NP* questions with 1 and 2 additional prepositional phrases (PPs). These embedded questions differ from the embedded questions in Experiment 1 only with regard to the length: embedded questions in Experiment 1 have the following structure: V + *who/which NP* question. In Experiment 3, however, this basic structure is extended by either 1 or 2 PPs inserted immediately after the *wh*-word and before the verb in embedded question.
4) Experiment 4: If there is a pattern in Croatian agrammatic aphasics' comprehension of active *who* vs. *which NP* dependencies, does it also exist in passivized *who/which NP* questions? This experiment tests for aphasics' comprehension of passivized *who which NP* questions.

All the experiments together contributed to answering General Question 2, as they all contained both *tko* "who" and *koji NP* "which NP" types of structures (with an exception of relative clauses – they contain only *koji* "which" structures).

6.4.2 Experiments

6.4.2.1 Experiment 1: Direct and Embedded *Who/Which NP* Questions, and Relative Clauses

Experiment 1 tested direct and embedded *who* and *which NP* subject-object questions, and subject-object relative clauses introduced by *which.* Experiment 1 is an act-out task. The experimenter acts out a scenario with toy animals and asks a question. Subjects are required to answer by pointing to one among 3 animals which they believe represents the correct answer. The participant and the experimenter would sit across the table, on which the toy animals were placed. The left-right orientation of toy animals was varied for the same reason pointed out by Smith & Mimica (1984), which is to avoid biased answers when there was a side preference, and also to prevent the participants from developing and following a strategy in answering the questions, instead of attending to the scenarios and questions.

There were always three animal figurines. Of these three animals, two that were identical "performed" the action expressed by a verb, such as *kissing* or *following*. For example, a giraffe, a tiger, and another giraffe would be lined up on the table, in that order. The experimenter would make the giraffe follow the tiger, and then the tiger would follow the other giraffe. The subject would then be asked the question: "Which giraffe followed the tiger?" and would be required to point to one of 3 animals. Above each question in the questionnaire, a scenario was written specifying who is following whom, and left or right direction of action was marked. Below each question the names of the three animals participating in the particular scenario were written, so that the experimenter could accurately mark the participant's answer. Only later the experimenter analysed the answers as correct or incorrect.

The experiment is a partial replication and adaptation of Thompson et al.'s (1999) experiment. Like Thompson et al.'s study, it contains direct *who/which NP* subject-object questions, but it does not test the questions with *what* and *which one* for semantic reasons. Since *what* in Croatian is used for inanimate objects, it would be odd to ask a question formed by "what" *što* (e.g., *Što je poljubilo žabu?* "What kissed the frog?"). Such a question sounds weird to a native speaker of Croatian, because an inanimate object is not capable of performing the action of kissing. Similarly, the sentential context required for *which one* in Croatian differs from the one in English. An expression semantically closest to *which one* in Croatian is *koji od njih,* while the semantics of *which one* is contained in *koji.*

The experiment contains the following 10 verbs: *slijediti* "follow", *ritnuti* "kick", *onjušiti* "sniff", *gurnuti* "push", *loviti* "chase", *poljubiti* "kiss", *dodirnuti* "touch", *ugristi* "bite", *preskočiti* "jump over", *liznuti* "lick". Since Croatian *koji NP* is marked for case, number and gender, Experiment 1 includes 4 masculine (*tigar* "tiger", *lav* "lion", *nosorog* "rhino", *nilski konj* "hyppo"), 4 feminine (*zebra* "zebra", *žirafa* "giraffe", *deva* "camel", *žaba* "frog") and 2 neuter (*lane* "fawn", *ždrijebe* "foal") nouns in singular. Plural was not tested in this study. The same verbs and nouns are used in Experiments 2 and 4.

The experiment contains 100 sentences: 10 subject and 10 object *who* and *which NP* direct questions (= 40), 10 subject and 10 object *who* and *which NP* embedded questions (= 40), and 10 subject and 10 object relative clauses introduced by *which* (= 20). Examples of stimuli in Experiment 1 are given in Table 6-4.1 below.

Table 6-4.1: Examples of stimuli in Experiment 1.

Sentence type	Examples of stimuli types
DQ-S-tko	Tko je lovio zebru? "Who chased the zebra?"
DQ-S-koji	Koja žirafa je preskočila zebru? "Which giraffe jumped over the zebra?"
DQ-O-tko	Koga je žirafa slijedila? "Who did the giraffe follow?"
DQ-O-koji	Koju zebru je žirafa gurnula? "Which zebra did the giraffe push?"
EQ-S-tko	Pokažite mi tko je slijedio žirafu. "Show me who followed the giraffe."
EQ-S-koji	Pokažite mi koja žirafa je preskočila zebru. "Show me which giraffe jumped over the zebra."
EQ-O-tko	Pokažite mi koga je žirafa slijedila. "Show me who the giraffe followed."
EQ-O-koji	Pokažite mi koju zebru je žirafa gurnula. "Show me which zebra the giraffe pushed."
RC-S-koji	Pokažite mi žirafu koja je ritnula zebru. "Show me the giraffe which kicked the zebra."
RC-O-koji	Pokažite mi žirafu koju je deva ritnula. "Show me the giraffe which the camel kicked."

6.4.2.2 Experiment 2: Long-Distance *Who/Which NP* Questions

The main goal of this experiment was to determine if there is a subject-object asymmetry in aphasics' comprehension of long-distance *tko* "who" and *koji NP* "which" NP questions. The experiment contains two versions of these questions. One version is represented by the long-distance subject-object *tko* and *koji NP* questions formed without the preposition *za*, while the other version of questions was formed with the preposition *za*. This experiment tests for aphasics' comprehension of syntactically complex *who/which NP* questions, looking for the asymmetry patterns.

Experiment 2 is also an act-out task. The same 10 verbs and same 10 nouns that were used in Experiment 1 were used in Experiment 2, but the nouns were assigned to different verbs. As in Experiment 1, there were always three animal figurines in a scenario, with two of them performing the same action. Actions were acted out by the experimenter, and subjects were required to point to an animal figurine as an answer to a particular question. The experimenter circled in the questionnaire the name of the animal to which the subject had pointed.

The experiment consists of 40 sentences: 10 subject and 10 object *who* questions (=20) and 10 subject and 10 object *which* NP questions (=20). Within each group of 10 questions, two forms were alternated: long-distance questions formed by a *wh*-word without the preposition *za* (*who/ which NP*) and constructions consisting of the preposition *za* and the *wh*-word (*who/which NP*).

Examples of stimuli used in Experiment 2 are presented in Table 6-4.2.

Table 6-4.2: Examples of stimuli used in Experiment 2.

Sentence type	Examples of stimuli types
LD-S-tko	Tko mislite da je ugrizao lava? "Who do you think bit the lion?"
LD-S-koji	Koji lav mislite da je lovio zebru? "Which lion do you think chased the zebru?"
LD-O-tko	Koga mislite da je lav preskočio? "Who do you think the lion jumped over?"
LD-O-koji	Koju žirafu mislite da je zebra gurnula? "Which giraffe do you think the zebra pushed?"
LD*za*-S-tko	Za koga mislite da je gurnuo žirafu? "Who do you think pushed the giraffe?"
LD*za*-S-koji	Za koju žirafu mislite da je slijedila zebru? "Which giraffe do you think followed the zebra?"
LD*za*-O-tko	Za koga mislite da ga je zebra gurnula? "Which giraffe do you think the zebra pushed?"
LD*za*-O-koji	Za koju zebru mislite da ju je deva gurnula? "Which zebra do you think the camel kicked?"

6.4.2.3 Experiment 3: Extended Embedded *Who/Which NP* Questions

This experiment was motivated by an ERP experiment described in Fiebach et al. (2002) that was conducted with healthy, adult German-speaking subjects. However, the version in the present study is a behavioral off-line experiment with Croatian–speaking aphasic population. The experiment exploits Fiebach et al.'s idea on intrasentential manipulation and increased sentence length as a test of WM in comprehension of embedded *wh*-questions.

The goal of the experiment was to determine whether increasing the distance between a displaced constituent (*who, which* NP) and its original position affects comprehension of embedded *tko* subject-object questions and embedded *koji NP* subject-object questions in Croatian aphasic patients. In Croatian, this type of intrasentential manipulation is easy to make due to its relatively free word order. Like German, Croatian has case endings that indicate the grammatical function of a word before the verb is encountered, which makes it a suitable candidate for experiments of this kind.

Table 6-4.3: Examples of stimuli in Experiment 3.

Sentence type	Examples of stimuli types
EQ1PP-S-tko	Petar zna tko je u utorak doktora zvao. "Peter knows who called the doctor on Tuesday."
EQ1PP-S-koji	Petar zna koji je pacijent u utorak doktora zvao. "Peter knows which patient called the doctor on Tuesday."
EQ1PP-O-tko	Petar zna koga je u utorak doktor zvao. "Peter knows who the doctor called on Tuesday."
EQ1PP-O-koji	Petar zna kojeg je pacijenta u utorak doktor zvao. "Peter knows which patient the doctor called on Tuesday."
EQ2PP-S-tko	Petar zna tko je u utorak iz javne govornice doktora zvao. "Peter knows who called the doctor from a telephone booth on Tuesday."
EQ2PP-S-koji	Petar zna koji je pacijent u utorak iz javne govornice doktora zvao. "Peter knows which patient called the doctor from a telephone booth on Tuesday."
EQ2PP–O-tko	Petar zna koga je u utorak iz javne govornice doktor zvao. "Peter knows who the doctor called from a telephone booth on Tuesday."
EQ2PP–O-koji	Petar zna kojeg je pacijenta u utorak iz javne govornice doktor zvao. "Peter knows which patient the doctor called from a telephone booth on Tuesday."

Note that embedded *who/which NP* questions in Experiment 1 are embedded questions formed as *Show me who/which NP* + V + N (e.g., *Show me which fawn kicked the frog*). Embedded questions in Experiment 3, however, have been extended to include 1 or 2 PPs (e.g. *Peter knows which fawn kicked the frog [by the river]*), *Peter knows which fawn kicked the frog [by the river][at dawn]*). The experiment consists of stimuli for: subject *tko*-questions with 1 extension (10), object *tko*-questions with 1 extension (10), subject *tko*-questions with 2 extensions (10), and object *tko*-questions with 2 extensions (10), subject *koji NP* questions with 1 extension (10), object *koji NP*-questions with 1 extension (10), subject *koji*

NP-questions with 2 extensions (10), and object *koji NP*-questions with 2 extensions (10).

In addition to 80 embedded *wh*-questions, Experiment 3 contains the same number of probe assertions for their verification. Each embedded question and the corresponding probe assertion were read once, with normal speed and intonation. The subjects were required to answer "Correct" if the probe assertation was correct, or "Incorrect" if the probe assertion was incorrect. The experimenter at the same time records the participiant's response by circling *T (Točno* "Correct"*)* or *N (Netočno* "Incorrect") on the questionnaire. Only after the experiment was completed did the experimenter compare subjects' answers with the correct answers that had been prepared in the Answer Key. *T* and *N* answers were compared with the answers in the Answer Key separately for each participant.

6.4.2.4 Experiment 4: Passivized *Who/ Which NP* Questions

The main purpose of this experiment was to determine if aphasic patients have difficulty understanding passivized *who/which NP* questions. A set of 20 passive sentences, 10 with the *by-phrase* and 10 without it, was administered as a pre-test. Testing for comprehension of passive sentences is relevant for comprehension of *which NP* questions, because the NP element in these questions undergoes the same syntactic transformation as passive sentences, i.e., NP movement. The experiment testing passivized *tko/koji NP* questions was motivated by Thompson et al.'s study (1999). Passivized *tko* and *koji NP* questions with a subject extraction are structurally parallel to English passive *who/which NP* questions (*Tko je praćen od zebre?* "Who was followed by the zebra?"). However, passivized *tko/koji NP* questions with an object gap in Croatian move the whole PP to the sentence initial position, while English leaves the *by* at the end (*Od koga je žirafa praćena?* "Who was the giraffe followed by?", and *Od kojeg lava je žirafa praćena?* "Which lion was the giraffe followed by?"). Thus, in English it involves extraction of the object of the preposition *by*. Since PP *za koga/za kojeg, u, e NP* is used to form long-distance questions and PP *od koga/od kojeg, -e, -eg NP* is used to form passivized questions, and given that these two types of questions employ two different types of movement, this experiment allows us to observe possible within and between case differences in realization of these syntactic operations. Again, a scenario was acted out by the experimenter and subjects were required to point to a correct animal figurine as an answer. Examples of stimuli used in this experiment are given in Table 6-4.4.

Table 6-4.4: Examples of stimuli used in Experiment 4.

Sentence type	Examples of stimuli types
PQ-S-tko	Tko je ritnut od žirafe? "Who was kicked by the giraffe?"
PQ-S-koji	Koja žirafa je slijeđena od lava? "Which giraffe was folloed by the lion?"
PQ-O-tko	Od koga je žirafa slijeđena? "Who was the giraffe followed by?"
PQ-O-koji	Od kojeg tigra je žirafa slijeđena? "Which tiger was the giraffe followed by?"

Thus, considering all structures in 4 experiments, each participant was tested on 30 types of *wh*-structures. The total number of tested sentences administered to each participant across the 4 experiments was 260, plus 80 probe assertions.

6.4.3 Experimental Sessions and Procedure

The tests and experiments presented above were distributed in 5 sessions that were administered over 4 weeks. The sentences from each experiment were first randomized in Excel and then divided into blocks. The blocks of randomized sentences from each experiment were further randomized. The experimental material was then divided into 5 sessions. Each experimental session was organized into 4 blocks, with short breaks between the blocks.

After obtaining a patient's signature as confirmation of their willingness to voluntarily participate in the study, the experimenter conducted an introductory session. The purpose of the introductory session was to allow the experimenter to collect enough information for making a decision on whether to continue testing and conduct experiments with the participant. The *Introductory session* consisted of *Elicited speech*, which was collected through informal exchange and description of *Cookie Theft* (Goodlgass & Kaplan, 1983), components of BDAE and selected *Supplementary tests*, as described in Section 6.3.3, *Digit Span* and the RCPM test, test of matching the animal names with the toys that would later be used in the experiments, and the pre-test sentences (Table 6-2).

All subjects were tested individually, in a quiet room. Each participant underwent testing in the same order of tests and received the same order of stimuli within the sessions. The participants were encouraged to stop at any point if they felt tired. Since the experiments focused not on how fast, but on how well aphasic patients can understand *wh*-dependencies, the participants were instructed to concentrate on the accuracy of their answers, and not on their speed in answering. Each session took approximately 50 to 60 minutes to complete. The experimenter explained all the tasks in detail, providing two trial examples for each type of *wh*-dependencies before testing commenced, whose purpose was to ensure that the participants understood the task. At the beginning of each session, the experimenter reminded the participants of the task instructions. Subjects were not given any feedback on the correctness of their responses during testing.

6.4.4 Statistics Used in Analysis of the Results of Experimental Measures

The likelihood of obtaining a certain score on the experimental measures was calculated by the binominal distribution test. As shown in Table 6-5, the tests differed in the value of n, the number of tested items, and p, the probability of obtaining a correct response. On the act-out tasks p =.333, as they all involve three toy animals, with one of the three representing the correct answer. On the tests with probe assertions p = .5, as the correct answer is either "Correct" or "Incorrect". The scores were then divided into three groups, depending on whether the probability of obtaining that particular score was greater/less than or equal to .05.

Table 6-5: Binominal probabilities for the experimental measures.

Experimental measure	*N*	*P*	Scores below chance	Scores at chance	Scores above chance
DQ	10	.333	0	1-6	7-10
EQ	10	.333	0	1-6	7-10
LD	5	.333	None	0-3	4-5
LD *za*	5	.333	None	0-3	4-5
EQ1PP	10	.5	0-2	3-7	8-10
EQ2PP	10	.5	0-2	3-7	8-10
PQ	10	.333	0	1-6	7-10
RC	10	.333	0	1-6	7-10

The Chi square test was further used to compare each individual's performance on subject vs. object extractions, and *tko* "who" vs. *koji NP* "which NP" dependencies. The results of all measures, evaluative and experimental, are presented in the next chapter.

6.5 Equipment and Supplies

Participants' elicited speech was tape-recorded on a *Sanyo* talk-book TRC 770M. A printed copy of the questionnaire was prepared for each session with each participant. It contained descriptions of scenarios, questions, and possible answers. The experimenter carefully followed the order of scenarios, marking the answers in the questionnaire.

Ten pairs of plastic toy animals were used for the act-out experiments. All animal figurines included in the experiments were brought to each session and used in tests with each participant. Several other toy animals, in addition to the basic set of 10 pairs, were brought to the *Introductory session*, because part of that session tested whether or not the participants could correctly match each toy animal used in experiments with its name.

CHAPTER SEVEN

EIGHT CASE STUDIES

In this chapter I present each of the eight aphasic patients in detail. Each case study consists of a brief description of lesion site and type of stroke, analysis of speech production based on the samples of spontaneous speech, and results of evaluative and experimental measures.

7.1 Case 1: S.T.

Ne mogu se sjetiti. "I can't remember." S.T.

S.T. is a 57-year-old right-handed female with 12 years of education and with a history of arterial hypertension. She had an ischemic stroke 9 months prior to her participation in this study. She was admitted to the hospital due to severe headache, numbness and weakness of the right limbs, severe disturbance of vision (the right eye) as well as motor and somatosensory disturbances. Additional symptoms in this patient included profound memory loss, speech disturbances, spatial disorientation, confusion and sleepiness. On examination, right hemianopia and the right-side facial paresis (the facial nerve (VII) was affected) were found. An MRI scan showed an ischemic infarct lesion in the left posterior cerebral artery (PCA). She was also diagnosed with the partial Gerstmann syndrome (dyslexia, dyscalculia) and aphasia. In addition, associative visual agnosia was present in this patient. This means that not only could she not recall names of objects, but she was also not able to name visually presented objects unless they were verbally described or unless she touched them.

The lesion site and the symptoms exhibited at the onset of disease, together with language related disturbancies she had shown, all indicate that she had had a transcortical sensory aphasia. However, at the time when the experiments were conducted for this study, her aphasia had reduced to anomia. At the moment of testing, apart from anomia, she exhibited other aberrations, such as semantic memory disturbances (e.g., difficulty remembering names of fruits, plants, cars, types of sports, and meanings of traffic signs), inability to fully understand conversation, or to sustain focus on the conversational topic. That this problem was not of exclusively linguistic nature supports the patient's observation:

> I can't do two things at the same time. I can't talk on the phone and write down a message. …when I exercise, if I spread my arms I forget to breathe. When I am in a group of people who are talking, I have to focus on one person only, and even then I can't understand everything.

7.1.1 S.T.'s Performance on Evaluative Measures

S.T.'s digit span was 8/14, and her performance on the RCPM was 34/36. Her performance on the portions on BDAE that tested comprehension and repetition was also very good. The results are summarized in the table below.

Table 7-1.1: S.T.'s scores on the subtests of BDAE.

BDAE Scores	
Word Discrimination (/72)	64
Body-Part Identification (/20)	20
Commands (/15)	15
Complex Ideational Material (/12)	10
Supplementary Language Tests	
Passive Subject-Object Discrimination (/5)	4
Indicative vs. Interrogative (/10)	10
Yes-No Questions (/5)	3
Wh-Questions (/5)	4

S.T. achieved a score of 10/10 on all 4 pre-tests of comprehension: simple declarative *netko,* passive *neki NP,* passive no-*by* and passive *by* sentences (Table 7.9).

7.1.2 S.T.'s Speech Characteristics

S.T.'s spontaneous speech is fluent, with good articulation and use of complex sentences, with occasional circumlocutions and semantic paraphasias. She produces sentences with a flat tone. During the first several months after her stroke, she was not able to sing, but at that time she was not aware of her flat tone: "I though I was singing, but I was only speaking." She is prone to losing the "thread" in communication, constructing incoherent discourse, which leaves impression that she is unable to follow Gricean principles of quantity and relevance in communication.

7.1.3 S.T.'s Performance on Experimental Measures

S.T. performed above chance on 29/30 different types of *wh*-structures. The only condition on which she did not perform above chance is embedded subject *which NP* questions with 2 PPs (see Table 7-10), but without a statistically significant subject-object difference. Raw scores for each experimental test are given in Table 7-10, and the percentages of *who* and *which* (*NP*) dependencies comprehended by S.T. are presented in Table 7-1.2.

Table 7-1.2: S.T.'s overall comprehension of *wh*-structures (percent correct).

S.T.	*Who*	*Which*	Total
Subject	98.3%	90%	94.6%
Object	88.3%	94.28%	91.53%
Total	93.3%	92.14%	92.6%

It is interesting that S.T. showed sentence comprehension at ceiling, given that often even after she correctly answered the questions, she still could not tell which toy represented which animal, unless she described them verbally or touched them. The fact that syntactic functioning, obviously facilitated by the inflectional system and other aspects of morphologically rich Croatian, is preserved while access to the lexicon is impaired in this patient indicates that there must be a mechanism connecting syntax to conceptual knowledge, which functions even when concepts fail to translate into words. More specifically, S.T. used a cognitive strategy that enabled her to integrate the mental representations necessary for comprehension, even though the representational devices failed to provide the necessary lexical knowledge, probably due to the patient's inability to temporally integrate the representations necessary for that lexical knowledge. Given the case-marking differences between subject and object *wh*-structures in Croatian, it is possible that S.T. relied on syntactic cueing (see Chpater 8). S.T.'s way of adjusting to her naming impairment is not unusual: various types of cueing as comprehension aid have been reported in the literature, such as prosodic (Strelnikov,

Vorobyev, Chernigovskaya & Medvedev, 2006), case cueing (Kempe & MacWhinney, 1999; Nagai et al., 2010), and other types of cueing (Silva-Pereyra, Conboy, Klarman & Kuhl, 2007).

7.2 Case 2: M.N.

Ne mogu govorit'. Ne mogu pisat' ni čitat'.
"Can't speak. Can't write or read." M.N.

A 48-year-old man, M.N., woke up one morning to find that he could not speak or use his right arm or leg. He was immediately transferred to a hospital where CT and MRI scans, together with the neurological examination, showed that he had just had an ischemic stroke. He was also diagnosed with Broca's aphasia. An MRI revealed a fronto-parietal post-insult lesion in the area supplied by the cortical branches of the left middle cerebral artery. The lesion was 4 x 3 x 4 cm, and located cortico-subcortially. Two chronic lacunar lesions were also found: one of them in the area of the left caput nuclei caudati and the other one in the area of the left putamen. The entire region showed local atrophic changes, with wider pericerebral subarachnoid liquor spaces, and a wider left lateral ventricle, especially in its frontal horn.

Over his 2-week stay at *Landesklinik Für Neurologie* in Salzburg[1], the hemiparesis in his right limbs became more discrete and, since his native language was not German, but Croatian, it was predicted that he would recover Croatian better than German. For that reason, it was recommended that he returns to Croatia for intensive speech therapy. After an intensive 3-week long treatment at a special hospital for medical rehabilitation in Croatia, the patient recovered from hemiparesis, but motor aphasia, alexia, agraphia, and acalculia were still present. Over the next 2 1/2 years the patient had been involved in speech therapy.

7.2.1 M.N.'s Performance on Evaluative Measures

M.N.'s score on the Digit Span was low, 2/14, while his performance on RCPM was high, 33/36. M.N.'s performance on the BDAE subtests was good; the results are presented in Table 7.2.1.

[1] The patient had lived in Germany for 6 years at the time he had a stroke.

Table 7-2.1: M.N.'s scores on the BDAE subtests.

BDAE Scores	
Word Discrimination (/72)	66
Body-Part Identification (/20)	19
Commands (/15)	15
Complex Ideational Material (/12)	11
Supplementary Language Tests	
Passive Subject-Object Discrimination (/5)	5
Indicative vs. Interrogative (/10)	10
Yes-No Questions (/5)	5
Wh-Questions (/5)	5

M.N.'s scores on the 4 pre-tests of comprehension are as follows: simple declarative *netko:* 9/10, passive *neki NP:* 7/10, passive no-*by*: 10/10 and passive *by* sentences: 10/10.

7.2.2 M.N.'s Speech Characteristics

The most prominent features of M.N.'s speech are nasalization of sounds, stuttering, distortions of phonemes and syllables, and paraphasias. Examples are given below.

1. ***Stuttering***
- *top-, top-, toplice* "spa",
- *probu-probu-probudio* "I woke up", followed by a sequence of 3-4 "uhms" before continuing the sentence.

2. ***Distortion of phonemes:***
- nasalization of sounds,
- ž > š *ženska* > *šenska* "woman".

3. ***Distortion of syllables***
- ao > o: *oti**šao*** > *o**šo*** "he left",
- ti > ø: *o**ti**šao* > *ošo,*
- pe > o: *petak* > *otak* "Friday",
- si> c: *declo* instead of *desilo* "happened",
- *žd* > *ž: Varaždinske Toplice* > *Varažinske Toplice* (toponim).

4. ***Circumlocutions***
- "homecountry": *Da se vrati u svoju ... đe mu je maternji jezik* "to return to his ... where his native language is spoken"

- "resident": *ova što radi da uči* "the one$_f$ who works to study".

5. Fillers:

- *Šta ja znam* "What do I know?"

6. Sentence structure

M.N.'s sentence is simple and often broken into fragments:

> *I kad su oni došli ja sam...a nisam nikako vidio... bilo je jedna šenska i ostalo su bili muškarci ... I oni su mene odatle ... ja njija čujem pa ne čujem... pa sam se probu-probu-probudio u 7 sati. Bio sam ... ležao sam u bolnici.*
>
> "[...] and when they came I was... and I coudn't see at all ... there were one female and the rest of them were males... And from there they ...me... I sort of hear them and then I don't ... so I wo-wo-woke up at 7 o'clock. I was ... I was lying at the hospital."

7. ***Agreement***

Occasionally, M.N. substitutes the participle ending for feminine *–la* by the particple ending for neuter *–lo:*

- *bi-**lo**$_{\text{lpt.sg.n.}}$. je [jedna šenska]$_{\text{Nom.sg.f.}}$* instead of: *bi-**la**$_{\text{lpt.sg.f.}}$ je jedna ženska* "there was one female".

7.2.3 M.N.'s Performance on Experimental Measures

M.N.'s performance on most of the conditions was above chance. However, that was not the case with his comprehension of embedded questions with 1 or 2 PPs (see Table 7-10). He performed at chance level on subject *who* embedded questions with 1 and 2 PPs, and on object *who* embedded questions with 2 PPs as well as on subject and object *which NP* embedded questions with 1 PP. However, no statistically significant differences in his comprehension of subject vs. object *who* and *which NP* structures in extended embedded questions were found.

Since the extensions in these questions add only to the length of sentences, and not to their complexity, and given M.N.'s low score on the Digit Span, it is not surprising that his comprehension of questions extended with 1 or 2 PPs was not as high as his scores on other syntactic tests. At the same time, his above chance comprehension on all other types of structures suggests that it is the memory load imposed by the extension of embedded questions that made his comprehension of these structures less successful. M.N.'s raw scores for each experimental test are given in

Table 7-10, and his overall percent correct answers are presented in Table 7-2.2.

Table 7-2.2: M.N.'s overall comprehension of *wh*-structures (percent correct).

M.N.	*Who*	*Which*	Total
Subject	81.6%	87.1%	84.6%
Object	93.3%	85.7%	89.2%
Total	87.5%	86.4%	87%

7.3 Case 3: P.J.

Riječi koje sam izbacivala je bilo perfektno!
"Words I was ejecting was perfect!" P.J.

A 57-year old female with a history of hypertension and ischemic stroke, P.J., was admitted to hospital due to a sudden loss of speech and weakness of the right limbs. Eight months earlier she had suffered an ischemic stroke, with infarction in the left lenticular nucleus extending up to the inferior horn of the lateral ventricle. The first stroke had caused the right-side hemiparesis and Broca's aphasia in the patient. She had recovered very well and several months later she even returned to work.

Apart from the old ischemic lesion in the basal ganglia, the MRI obtained after the second cerebrovascular accident showed obliteration of both the left internal carotid (ICA) and the left middle cerebral artery (MCA). In addition, stenosis (narrowing) of the left anterior communicating artery (ACA) was found. The left lateral ventricle was wider than the right one, due to post-insult changes. In this patient, a type of vasculopathy known as Moya-Moya, causing degenerative changes of ICA and MCA and channeling the blood flow towards the smaller vessels, had caused the second ischemic stroke. This stroke had left the patient, P.J., with a more profound aphasia than the first stroke as well as with a slight right-side hemiparesis.

7.3.1 P.J.'s Performance on Evaluative Measures

P.J.'s score on the Digit Span was 4/14, and on RCPM 31/36. Like S.T. and M.N., she performed well on the comprehension subtests. Her performance on the BDAE subtests is summarized in Table 7-3.1.

Table 7-3.1: P.J.'s scores on BDAE subtests.

BDAE Scores	
Word Discrimination (/72)	64
Body-Part Identification (/20)	19
Commands (/15)	14
Complex Ideational Material (/12)	8
Supplementary Language Tests	
Passive Subject-Object Discrimination (/5)	5
Indicative vs. Interrogative (/10)	10
Yes-No Questions (/5)	5
Wh-Questions (/5)	5

Like S.T.'s, P.J.'s scores on all the 4 pre-tests of comprehension (simple declarative *netko,* passive *neki NP,* passive no-*by*, and passive *by* sentences) are 10/10.

7.3.2 P.J.'s Speech Characteristics

There are two prominent characteristics of P.J.'s spontaneous speech: stuttering and insertion of a semivowel in combinations of sounds that she finds difficult.

1. Stuttering:

- *sa-sa-sa-sa-sa-sa … ovaj engleskim hm- hm- hm- …nakon toga predivno je bilo mu-mu-mu kaj sam ja naučila taj engleski!*
"with- with-with….. …. … …this… English …huh…. .. . after that it was wonderful him-him-him that I learnt English!"
- *ot-ot-otpelali* instead of *otpelali* (Kaikavism) "drove away",
- *Engleski je pre-pre-prevladavao na svim poljima* "English was predominant in all domains".

2. Epenthesis

P.J. inserts an epenthetic sound, a semivowel (marked as ь in the examples below) systematically before every "r" in a word, and occasionally in other positions:

- *stьrašno* "aweful", *pьrekьrasno* "wonderful", *Kьrapinske* (toponim), *kьrevet* "bed"; *tьrinaestoga tьrećega* "March 13th"; *pьrobudila* "woke up";
- *kьćer* "daughter", *dьva* "two" *sьve* "all",
- after p and f: *pьosao* "work", *fьotelja* "armchair".

It is possible that this is P.J.'s strategy for facilitating pronunciation of words that she finds difficult. This strategy is often used by Broca's aphasics (Goodglass, 1993).

3. Agreement

P.J. overuses the endings that mark neuter. Examples in which she used the endings for neuter instead of endings for masculine are:

- *Engleski*$_{m}$ *mi je bi*-lo$_{\text{lpt.sg.n}}$ *lak-o*$_{n}$ instead of *Engleski mi je bi-o*$_{\text{lpt.sg.m.}}$ *lak* "English was easy to me",
- *Moj*$_{m}$ *rječnik*$_{m}$ *u engleskom je bolj-e*$_{n}$ *nego u hrvatskom!* instead of: *Moj rječnik u engleskom je bolj-i*$_{m}$ *nego u hrvatskom!* "My vocabulary is better in English than in Croatian",

She also uses the neuter markings instead of feminine endings:

- *Kćer*$_{f.}$ *moja*$_{f}$ *u tome krevetu spavalo*$_{\text{lpt.sg.n.}}$ instead of Kćer$_{\text{f.}}$ moja$_{\text{f.}}$ je u tome krevetu spavala$_{\text{lpt.sg.f.}}$ "My daugther slept in that bed."
- *Znam da se probudilo*$_{\text{lpt.sg.n.}}$ ... *nelagoda*$_{g.f}$ instead of: *Znam da me je probudila*$_{\text{lpt.sg.f}}$ *nelagoda*. "I know that a feeling of discomfort woke me up."
- *Riječi*$_{\text{Nom.pl.f.}}$ *koje* $_{\text{Nom.pl.f.}}$ *sam izbacivala je*$_{\text{Aux3sg.pres.}}$ *bilo*$_{\text{lpt.sg.n.}}$ *perfektno*$_{n}$, *perfektno!* instead of: *Riječi koje* $_{\text{Nom.pl.f}}$ *sam izbacivala*$_{\text{lpt.sg.f.}}$ *bile*$_{\text{lpt.pl.f.}}$ *su*$_{\text{Aux2pl.pres}}$ *perfektne* $_{Nom.pl.f}$ "Words I was ejecting were perfect, perfect!"

4. Omissions

P.J. omits auxiliary verbs, as in:

- *Kćer moja u tome krevetu spavalo,* instead of: *Kćer moja je u tome krevetu spavala,*

and omits or substitutes personal pronouns, for instance the clitic *me* "I$_{\text{Acc}}$" in:

- *Znam da se probudilo... nelagoda,* instead of: *Znam da me je probudila nelagoda.*

5. Prepositions

Occasionally P.J. fails to use a correct case ending on a noun required by a preposition, as in:

- *Ne znam kako sam došla do fotelja*$_{\text{Nom}}$ [correct form: *do fotelje*$_{\text{Gen}}$] "I don't know how I got to the armchair".

She also leaves out the preposition if it begins with the same sound as the word which follows the preposition, as in:

- *Fiona došla svojim mužem Irske*, instead of: *Fiona došla sa svojim mužem iz Irske.* "Fiona arrived with her husband from Ireland."

It is possible that the first preposition *sa* “with” is left out due to reduction to its shorter form, *s,* which then assimilated with the *s* belonging to the possessive pronoun *svojim.* Since the short form of the preposition would be incorrect in this context, given that the next word, *svojim,* begins with the same consonant, which makes it difficult to pronounce, a prescriptive orthographic and orthoepic rule in Croatian prohibits such shortening. Since the use of the shorter form in this context and assimilation of two *s* lead to elimination of the preposition, this is probably an agrammatic feature. Leaving out the second preposition, *iz* “from”, can be interpreted only as a feature of agrammatism.

7.3.3 P.J.’s Performance on Experimental Measures

P.J. comprehended 78.5% of *wh*-dependencies tested in 4 experiments (Table 7-3.2). Her comprehension of extended embedded *who* questions was like M.N.’s: above chance comprehension of object questions, but chance comprehension of subject questions, and chance level comprehension of both subject and object embedded *which NP* questions with 1 PP. She also comprehended embedded subject *which NP* questions at chance level. However, there were no statistically significant differences in P.J.’s comprehension of subject-object *who* and *which NP* extended embedded questions.

Another type of *wh*-dependencies that P.J. comprehended at chance level are subject and object passivized *who* questions, again without statistically significant differences (as a matter of fact, the raw scores for subject and object questions on this condition were identical, as shown in Table 7-10). P.J.’s chance comprehension of subject and object passivized *who* questions is surprising, given that her comprehension of passive structures without *wh*-constituents was flawless (see Table 7-9). Thus, the difference is probably not caused by a passive structure as such, but rather by something else, related to the nature of *who* in a passivized context. This conclusion is further supported by the fact that her comprehension of passivized subject and object *which NP* questions was above chance. Furthermore, the passivized questions are the only type of *wh*-dependencies on which P.J.’s comprehension of both subject and object *who*-dependencies was at chance, while her comprehension of both subject and object *which NP*-dependencies was above chance. In addition, her performance on the BDAE subtest *Passive Subject-Object Discrimination* was at ceiling. It is possible, then, that for P.J. morphologically less specified *who* was harder to comprehend in the passivized context.

However, the difference in her comprehension of *who* vs. *which* NP passivized questions was not statistically significant.

In short, this patient did not display any statistically significant differences in comprehension of subject vs. object *who/which NP* dependencies.

Table 7-3.2: P.J.'s overall comprehension of *wh*-structures (percent correct).

P.J.	*Who*	*Which*	Total
Subject	75%	77.14%	76.15%
Object	81.6%	80%	80.76%
Total	78.3%	78.57%	78.5%

7.4 Case 4: AD

Teško govorim. "It's hard (for me) to speak." A.D.

A 77-year-old hypertensive, right-handed female, A.D., who was hospitalized for urosepsis, suddenly lost her ability to speak and experienced right-side central facial paresis as well as weakness of the left arm. She was immediately transferred to the Neurological Clinic, where a CT scan together with neurological examination as well as progress of the disease indicated ischemic cerebral stroke. The second CT scan confirmed signs of vascular encephalopathy and the ultrasound examination of the patient's head and neck vasculature showed diffuse atherosclerotic changes, with stenosis at the origin of both internal carotid arteries (ICAs). She was also diagnosed with Broca's aphasia.

7.4.1 A.D.'s Performance on Evaluative Measures

A.D. achieved only 2/14 on the Digit Span, and 27/36 on the RCPM test. Her performance on the BDAE subtests was relatively good, as shown in Table 7-4.1.

Table 7-4.1: A.D.'s scores on the BDAE subtests.

BDAE Scores	
Word Discrimination (/72)	71
Body-Part Identification (/20)	20
Commands (/15)	12
Complex Ideational Material (/12)	10
Supplementary Language Tests	
Passive Subject-Object Discrimination (/5)	4
Indicative vs. Interrogative (/10)	8
Yes-No Questions (/5)	3
Wh-Questions (/5)	4

Like S.T. and P.J., A.D. scored 10/10 on all the 4 pre-tests of comprehension (simple declarative *netko,* passive *neki NP,* passive no-*by*, and passive *by* sentences).

7.4.2 A.D.'s Speech production

A.D.'s spontaneous speech is fluent, but slowed and to some extent slurred. She exhibits signs of dysarthria. Note that her deficit, probably best characterized as mild, is *phonetic*, consisting of acoustic aberration of speech, and not *phonemic*, which means impairment of selection and ordering of phonemes. A.D. does not use phonemic and semantic paraphasias, or neologisms. She does not delete or substitute bound morphemes, and correctly matches inflectional endings in a sentence. A.D. does not leave out prepositions, conjunctions or other function words, although she shows occasional word-finding difficulties with regard to content words, which slows down her speech production.

A.D. produces well-formed, usually not very long but sometimes complex sentences, such as relative clauses. This sentence is an example from her description of the *Cookie Theft* picture:

(1) *Ova slika prikazuje domaćicu u kuhinji kako briše tanjur.*
"This picture presents a housewife in a kitchen who is wiping a plate."

Although she leaves the impression that her comprehension of conversation is good, she often asks the experimenter to repeat the experimental questions or task instructions. This can be caused by her difficulty to focus on the conversational topic rather than a comprehension deficit, given that her comprehension in conversation appears intact. Since the problematic features of A.D.'s speech are related to articulation, without signs of breakdown of grammatical relations in speech production, the conclusion is that this Broca's aphasic is not agrammatic.

7.4.3 A.D.'s Performance on Experimental Measures

On most tests A.D. performed above chance. However, like M.N. and P.J., she showed difficulty comprehending extended embedded questions formed by either *who* or *which NP* – these questions she comprehended at chance level. Her comprehension of passivized *who* questions was at ceiling. She comprehended passivized subject *which NP* questions above chance, but her comprehension of passivized *which NP* object questions was at the chance level. However, no statistically significant subject-object differences were found in her comprehension of *wh*-dependencies.

Table 7.4.2: A.D.'s overall comprehension of *wh*-structures (percent correct).

A.D.	*Who*	*Which*	*Total*
Subject	81.6%	78.57%	80%
Object	83.3%	80%	81.5%
Total	82.5%	79.28%	80.7%

While there were no statistically significant subject-object differences in her comprehension results, there was 1 statistically significant *who-which NP* difference, indicating that A.D. comprehended better *who* than *which NP* passivized questions with object extractions ($\chi^2(1) = 5.000$, $p = .0253 < .05$).

7.5 Case 5: T.P.

Ne mogu... govorit. "Can't ... speak." T.P.

A 52-year-old man with history of hypertension, T.P., was admitted to the Neurological Clinic due a sudden loss of speech and profound motoric deficit of the right limbs. Paresis of the right hypoglossal (XII) and facial (VII) nerves were also present. A CT scan and Transcranial Doppler ultrasound examination showed an occlusion of the left internal carotid artery (ICA) at the origin, and stenosis of the right ICA at the origin of 40%. Infarction had left a 3 x 2 cm cortico-subcortical ischemic lesion. A Transcranial Doppler examination revealed asymmetric circulation of the

Willis circle and the formation of a collateral path due to zero circulation in the left external carotid artery (ECA). In addition, the left Sylvian fissure and the left temporo-parietal sulci were narrower, and the left parietal sulci were more attenuated. An ischemic stroke caused a mixed nonfluent aphasia in this patient, and left him with a significant motor difficulty in the left limbs.

7.5.1 T.P.'s Performance on Evaluative Measures

T.P. achieved a score of 5/14 on the Digit Span, and 22/36 on the RCPM. Note that his RCPM score was the lowest within the range of scores for all Broca's and mixed nonfluent cases of aphasia (22-34), being higher only than the score achieved by the patient with mixed fluent aphasia, whose score was 16/36. T.P.'s relatively low score on the RCPM is surprising, if we accept the hypothesis that language and intelligence are separate cognitive systems. However, his relatively low score on the non-verbal intelligence test may have been caused by changes on the ICAs (occlusion of the left ICA and stenosis of 40% of the right ICA).

T.P.'s performance on the BDAE subtests of comprehension was slightly worse than P.J.'s performance. Although he achieved 10/10 on repetition of indicative vs. interrogative structures, he achieved only 4/10 on asking questions. His comprehension of passive structures tested by the BDAE *Passive Subject-Object Discrimination* subtest was very good, as shown in Table 7-5.1. Thus, one could expect good comprehension of passive structures, but some difficulties in comprehension of *wh*-constructions. The results on the BDAE subtests are summarized in Table 7-5.1.

Table 7-5.1: T.P.'s scores on BDAE subtests.

BDAE Scores	
Word Discrimination (/72)	62
Body-Part Identification (/20)	18
Commands (/15)	9
Complex Ideational Material (/12)	9
Supplementary Language Tests	
Passive Subject-Object Discrimination (/5)	4
Indicative vs. Interrogative (/10)	10
Yes-No Questions (/5)	2
Wh-Questions (/5)	2

T.P.'s scores on the 4 pre-tests of comprehension are: simple declarative *netko:* 7/10, passive *neki NP:* 7/10, passive no-*by*: 6/10, and passive *by* sentences: 9/10.

7.5.2 T.P.'s Speech Characteristics

T.P.'s speech is forced, reduced to few words with distorted syllables and phonemes. His articulation is impaired, due to impairment of the hypoglossal nerve, which innervates the muscles of the tongue. His speech is also hypophonic, i.e., his voice volume is reduced. T.P. produces paraphasias, but neologisms are not typical for his speech. Examples of his speech errors include:

1. Distortion of phonemes
- h > ø: *kuinja* instead of *kuhinja* "kitchen"; *ovi dana,* instead of: *ovih dana* "these days",
- s > c: *docta,* instead of: *dosta* "enough",
- ž > š: *žena* > *šena* "woman".

2. Distortion of syllables
- *tiše* > *briše* "wipe$_{3.sg.pres.}$"

3. Epenthesis (r)
- *ova šena ršiše tanjur,* instead of: *ova žena briše tanjur* "this woman is wiping a plate".

4. Paraphasia
- *kolac* "stick", instead of: *stolac* "chair".

5. Grammar
T.P. correctly uses tenses, possessive construction *od + Genitive,* and cases, as illustrated by the following examples:
- *Imam*$_{1sg.pres}$ *šenu*$_{Acc}$, *ćer*$_{Acc}$...*ovaj... ovo je majka*$_{Nom}$ *od šene*$_{Gen}$... *ovo je mala*$_{Nom}$ "I have a wife, a daugther...this... this is my wife's mother... this is the little one [girl]";
- *Ka ću ja moći...ovaj...uh!* when AUX$_{1sg.fut.}$I may "When will I be able to... this...uh!"

7.5.3 T.P.'s Performance on Experimental Measures

Overall, T.P. comprehended 70.3% of *wh*-dependencies tested in this study (Table 7-5.2). T.P. comprehended direct subject and object *who* and *which NP* questions above chance. His comprehension of subject and object long-distance *who* and *which NP* questions with and without the preposition *za* was also above chance, with the exception of subject *who* questions with *za*, where he performed at chance level. T.P.'s comprehension of embedded questions with 1 and 2 PPs was at chance, while his comprehension of passivized questions as well as relative clauses was above chance. Statistical analyses have revealed 1 statistically significant subject-object difference in T.P.'s comprehension of embedded *who* questions ($\chi^2(1) = 6.667, p = .0098 < .05$), with better comprehension of object than subject extractions, and no significant *who-which NP* differences.

Table 7-5.2: T.P.'s overall comprehension of *wh*-structures (percent correct).

T.P.	*Who*	*Which*	Total
Subject	66.6%	63.3%	66.1%
Object	76.6%	71.6%	74.6%
Total	71.6%	69.28%	70.38%

7.6 Case 6: B.R.

On zabrza, pa sve pom'ješa.
"He speeds up, and mixes up everything". B.R.'s wife

B.R. is a 59-year-old male with 14 years of education. During the period of nine years before his illness, he worked in Germany from time to time and become fluent in German. He participated in this study 15 months after he had a stroke. B.R. had suffered from hypertension and cardiopathy for several years prior his stroke, but he did not regularly take the medications prescribed for his illness. One morning he experienced a sudden weakness of the right limbs and had difficulty speaking. On admission to the hospital, a CT scan showed a big intracerebral hematoma in the left basal ganglia as well as a wider left lateral ventricle and its frontal horn. On admission, the right side hemiparesis and motor aphasia were dominant. After a two-week stay at the hospital, he was transferred to a special hospital for medical rehabilitation, where he stayed for 6 weeks. After that, he started speech therapy at SUVAG, where he was seen on a weekly basis by a speech pathologist, who at that time found that B.R. had a mixed nonfluent aphasia. Note that the type of stroke he had had (intracerebral hemorrhage) differs from the type of stroke in the 7 remaining aphasic participants in this study, who all had had ischemia.

7.6.1 B.R.'s Performance on Evaluative Measures

B.R.'s digit span was extremely low: 1/14. His score on the RCPM was 25/36. His scores on the BDAE subtests were much lower than the scores of other participants presented above. He performed much better on subtests pertaining to auditory word comprehension, while his score on the subtest *Passive Subject-Object Discrimination* was 1/5. He showed difficulty forming questions, too. The scores of his performance on the BDAE subtests are presented in Table 7-6.1.

Table 7-6.1: B.R.'s scores on the BDAE subtests.

BDAE Scores	
Word Discrimination (/72)	45.5
Body-Part Identification (/20)	16
Commands (/15)	6
Complex Ideational Material (/12)	10
Supplementary Language Tests	
Passive Subject-Object Discrimination (/5)	1
Indicative vs. Interrogative (/10)	4
Yes-No Questions (/5)	1
Wh-Questions (/5)	2

B.R.'s scores on the 4 pre-tests of comprehension are as follows: simple declarative *netko:* 8/10, passive *neki NP:* 9/10, passive no-*by*: 3/10, and passive *by* sentences: 7/10.

7.6.2 B.R.'s Speech Characteristics

At the time of testing, B.R. showed many symptoms of Broca's aphasia: nonfluent speech, reduced to short phrases, paraphasias, circumlocutions, and impaired intra-sentential relations. His motor agility was also impaired: his right arm was almost completely nonfunctional, and although his right leg was more functional than his right arm, he used a cane for walking. Due to right-side facioparesis and bucco-facial apraxia,

B.R.'s articulation is limited and slurred. In addition, his speech is excessively rapid. Since these characteristics are often combined with phonemic and semantic paraphasias in his speech, it all results in an unintelligible speech output. In addition, B.R.'s voice volume is pathologically reduced, i.e., it is hypophonic. Hypophonia often accompanies aphasia secondary to deep subcortical lesions, such as deep anterior lesions involving the basal ganglia (Goodlgass, 1993). B.R.'s conversational ability is seriously impaired, manifested as an inability to function as a hearer, due to his efforts to echo the speaker's words (echolalia) or because B.R. interrupts the speaker. This may be caused by a reduced attention span. Finally, his language breakdown is cross-modal, manifested also as dyslexia and dyscalculia.

Examples of B.R.'s speech errors are given below.

1. Distortions of phonemes

- m > p: *piljama* instead of *miljama* "for miles",
- l > lj: before *i: pljiva* instead of *pliva* "swim",
- d > č: *čječaka* instead of *dječaka* "boy$_{\text{Gen-Acc}}$",
- h > ø: *rvacki* instead of *hrvatski* "Croatian",
- ts > c: *rvacki* instead of *hrvatski* "Croatian",
- s > c: *cudoper* instead of *sudoper* "sink",
- d > b: *cvodi* instead of *sobi* "room",
- closing of the vowel *o > u: uvaj je unoga...* instead of *ovaj je onoga...* "this one [did something to] that one".

2. Distortions of syllables

- že > še: *može > moše* "may$_{\text{3sg.pres.f/m/n.}}$", but also:
- *šoše* instead of *može* "may$_{\text{3s.pres. f/m/n.}}$",
- *šiši* instead of *kiši* "it is raining",
- *tatedrala* instead of *katedrala* "cathedral",
- *lavaći* instead of *lajati* "to bark".

3. Paraphasias

- *krokodil* "crocodile" instead of *nilski konj* "hippo",
- *katkus* instead of *kaktus,*
- *htjela* "want$_{\text{3.sg.f.past}}$" instead of *želi* "wish$_{\text{3.s.f / m.pres.}}$" – here not only he substituted words, but also verb's tense: instead of present, he used past participle, but he correctly chose the ending *–la* to encode the feminine gender.

4. Circumlocutions

- *ona ... što je jača* "the [animal] that is stronger" for "lion".

5. Prepositions

B.R. correctly uses prepositions, as shown in the PPs below.

- *u cvodi* instead of *u sobi* "at the room",
- *kod kuće* "at home".

The case endings on the nouns following the prepositions are also correctly used; for instance, Locative endings, as shown above, and Genitive ending, as in:

- *od motora* "by the motorbike".

6. Agreement

- *Neko vadi neke*$_{\text{Acc.pl.f.}}$ ... *voće*$_{\text{Acc.n}}$.

In this example, instead of choosing the Accusative ending *–o* for *neko,* which needs to agree with the collective noun in neuter *voće* "fruits" (Nominative: *voće*, Genitive: *voća,* Dative: *voću*, Accusative: *voće*, etc.), B.R. chose the Accusative ending *-e*, which is correct if used for a feminine noun in singular, like voćka$_{\text{Nom.s.f.}}$, but he did not choose that noun. Thus, the substitution of bound morpheme was realized within the same category (gender) and it followed the markedness principle in allowing the more prominent element—feminine—to replace the less pronounced element of the same category—neuter.

7. Omissions

Although in spontaneous speech B.R. overuses demonstrative pronouns (e.g., *ovaj, onaj,* "this", "that"), a prediction that his use of pronouns in general is intact is wrong: he omits personal pronouns in oblique cases, especially when they take a form of clitic in Accusative.

- *udari ... ako plače* instead of *udari* ***ga***$_{\text{Acc.m.}}$ *ako plače* "slap him if he cries",
- *nahrani ... ako plače* instead of *nahrani* ***ju***$_{\text{Acc.f.}}$ *ako plače* "feed her if she cries".

Another interesting type of omission is found in examples such as:

- *moše pliva piljama* instead of *može plivati miljama* "he can swim for miles".

Omission of the infinitive ending *–ti* leaves the verb form as *pliva-ø*, with the zero morpheme, which marks 3rd person singular of the present tense. However, the auxiliary verb *moći* in the construction above requires either infinitive (*može plivati*), which is typical for Croatian, or the construction consisting of *da* (Comp) + present (e.g., *može da pliva*), which is typical for the Serbian language. Even if B.R. wanted to use the construction *da + present* (*da pliva*), he omitted the complementizer *da.* In a study with Serbian fluent aphasics, Kljajevic and Bastiaanse (2011) have shown that these speakers exhibited a pattern of systematic substitution of the infinitival constructions with the present tense in 22.9% of cases and with the *da + present* construction in 4.1% of cases. Omission of the ending *–ti* in infinitive *plivati* "to swim" changes this verb form into the 3rd person present tense form *pliva* "(he/she) swims", with the correct ending for the 3rd person singular present tense, which is the ø-morpheme, just like in the modal verb *moći – može.* Note that, even though they both have the ø-morpheme ending, the 3rd person singular of the modal verb *moći* (*može*) and *plivati* (*pliva*) do not coincide in form. This indicates that B.R. did not simply leave out a bound morpheme or copied the form or ending of the 3rd person present of the modal verb in producing the main verb. Instead, he applied a rule of grammar that requires the ø-morpheme to be added to the correct infinitival stem. Thus, although it appears that B.R. omitted a bound morpheme, this error was not an omission but rather a substitution error, which was made in accordance with the rules of grammar (see Section 2.4.1 for similar examples from German and Polish). Finally, the example does not indicate difficulty with time reference, because the construction *može plivati/ da pliva miljama* refers to the present, and B.R. substituted the construction with the present tense. This means that the substitution error was within the same time frame (i.e., both verb forms refer to the present) and suggests that combining a modal verb in the present tense with the main verb in infinitive was too difficult for B.R.

7.6.3 B.R.'s Performance on Experimental Measures

There were 12 statistically significant differences in B.R.'s comprehension of *who* and *which NP* dependencies: 10 indicate a subject-object asymmetry and 2 indicate a *who-which NP* asymmetry.

7.6.3.1 Subject-Object Asymmetries in B.R.'s Comprehension

From the 10 statistically significant subject-object differences in B.R.'s comprehension of the tested *wh*-dependencies, 5 indicated better comprehension of object, and 3 indicated better comprehension of subject structures. Better comprehension of object extractions was found in his comprehension of direct *who* questions ($\chi^2(1) = 5.495$, $p = .0196 < .05$), long distance *who* questions ($\chi^2(1) = 4.286$, $p = .0384 < .05$), embedded *who* questions ($\chi^2(1) = 5.495$, $p = .0196 < .05$), direct *which NP* questions ($\chi^2(1) = 7.500$, $p = .0062 < .05$), long distance *which NP* questions ($\chi^2(1) = 6.667$, $p = .0098 < .05$), embedded *which NP* questions ($\chi^2(1) = 5.495$, $p = .0191 < .05$), and relative clauses ($\chi^2(1) = 8.571$, $p = .0034 < .05$). It is interesting that his pattern of comprehension of passive questions ran in the opposite direction, with better comprehension of subject than object structures both in passivized *who* ($\chi^2(1) = 5.495$, $p = .0196 < .05$) and *which NP* questions $\chi^2(1) = 13.333$, $p = .0003 < .05$). This pattern is discussed in Chapter 8.

7.6.3.1.1 Direct *who/which NP* questions

B.R. comprehended direct object *who* questions above chance, but direct subject questions below chance. Note that the same pattern was also found in his comprehension of *which NP* questions. A possible explanation of these data relies on the morphological features of *tko, koji* and their contribution to sentence processing. As discussed in Chapter 5, morphological case can facilitate comprehension processes by triggering predictions on the grammatical and thematic roles in a sentence. For example, the Accusative ending suggests the grammatical role of a direct object, Nominative suggests the role of subject, while Dative suggests the role of indirect object. As soon as a prediction of grammatical role is made, a prediction of thematic role can follow. Thus, direct objects are usually associated with Patient, while subjects can be associated with many more thematic roles: Agent, Beneficiary, Source, Theme, etc. Although these thematic roles may obey some hierarchical principle in being assigned to the nouns with the grammatical function of subject, it still may be difficult to choose from all the possible options, i.e., to correctly predict thematic role of a particular constituent marked by Nominative (the roles are checked against the verb once it is encountered). This results in better comprehension of object than subject *wh*-questions. It seems that, at least in the case of B.R., this happens in all types of *wh*-dependencies, except those that require more processing resources, like extended embedded questions, or in structures that require another strategy for comprehension, such as passivized questions.

7.6.3.1.2 Long-distance *who/which NP* questions

B.R. comprehended all object structures in long-distance questions above chance. Above chance comprehension of long-distance dependencies with the preposition *za* is probably facilitated by the presence of the resumptive pronoun.

(2) Za koga$_i$ mislite da *ga$_i$* je zebra pratila t$_i$?
for who think$_{2.pl.pres.}$ that he$_{Acc}$ AUX$_{3sg.pres.}$ zebra follow$_{lpt.sg.f.}$
"Who do you think the zebra followed?"

Even when the resumptive pronoun is not present, B.R. comprehends long-distance object questions.

(3) Koga$_i$ mislite da je zebra pratila t$_i$?
who think$_{2.pl.pres}$ that AUX$_{3sg.pres.}$ zebra follow$_{lpt.sg.f.}$
"Who do you think the zebra followed?"

His comprehension of subject structures within long-distance dependencies was poor, with the exception of long-distance *who* questions with the preposition *za.* A statistically significant subject-object asymmetry, with above chance comprehension of object structures, was found in long-distance *who* and *which NP* questions without the preposition *za.* Since extraction from subject position in embedded questions happens in Croatian, the question is: How to explain their grammaticality?

Sentences such as (4) violate the ECP, according to which traces must be properly governed, either theta-governed or antecedent-governed.

(4) Tko$_i$ mislite t' da t$_i$ je pratio zebru?
who$_{Nom}$ think$_{2pl.pres}$ that Aux$_{3sg.pres.}$ follow$_{lpt.sg.m.}$ zebra$_{Acc}$
"Who do you think followed the zebra?"

Since the complementizer *da* "that" blocks government, the trace is not properly governed and, according to GB, the sentence is ungrammatical. Its English counterpart is also considered ungrammatical, as shown in (5) (where the star indicates ungrammaticality of the sentence).

(5) *Who do you think that t followed the zebra?

However, (5) was acceptable in Old and Middle English, and the same *type* of structure is acceptable in other languages, such as Norwegian. Given the lack of a workable solution to this problem at the moment, and since *that t* seems to be a question of parametric variation, and not of grammaticality/ungrammaticality in terms of violating/not violating UG, we can only conclude that the structures such as (4) are not necessarily ungrammatical in Croatian[2].

7.6.3.1.3 Embedded *who/which NP* questions

B.R.'s comprehension of object extractions was better than his comprehension of subject extractions in *who/ which NP* direct, embedded, and long-distance questions without the presposition *za*, as well as in relative clauses. However, this pattern does not hold for his comprehension of extended embedded and passivized questions. Actually, a reverse pattern appears in his comprehension of extended embedded *who* questions with 1 PP. The same trend is observed in his comprehension of embedded *which NP* questions with 1 PP, but the difference does not reach statistical significance in this case. While his comprehension of embedded *who* questions with 2 PPs is above chance, his comprehension of embedded *which NP* with 2 PPs is at chance.

In order to analyze the difference in the two patterns, it is necessary to briefly discuss the task in Experiment 3. In this experiment, extended embedded questions were tested in a verification paradigm with probe assertions. Each probe assertion consists of a simple declarative sentence, whose meaning is always contained in the embedded questions they test, and varied only for truth or falsity by either matching the subject and object of a probe assertion with the subject and object of the embedded question, in which case the assertion is true, or by not matching them, in which case the assertion is false. Since the meaning of probe assertions is always contained in embedded questions they test, in order to arrive at a correct judgement of probe assertions, a person needs to construct syntactic representations of both embedded questions and probe assertions, compare their subject and object positions, and based on this comparison decide whether the representation of probe assertion semantically matches the representation of the embedded question or not.

A task with similar demand is contained in the BDAE subtests—*Passive Subject-Object Discrimination*: a subject is required to listen to a sentence and answer a question pertaining to it, but a correct answer can be obtained only by comparing subject and object positions in the syntactic representation of the declarative sentence and the *wh*-question. Here is an example from that subtest:

---

[2] Consider the fact that Croatian also violates the principle of constituent dependency, which is one of the basic principles of UG. In the sentence: *Markov ti prijatelj šalje pozdrav* "Mark's friend is sending you his regards", the constituent *Markov prijatelj* is disrupted by the clitic *ti*.

(6) “If I told you: ‘The lion was killed by the tiger’, which animal is dead?”

This example contains three structures (conditional, passive, and a *wh*-question), which make it complex and in terms of processing a demanding sentence. In order to arrive at a correct answer, a patient needs to construct syntactic representations of the passive sentence and *wh*-question, and compare them.

Experiment 3 requires a comparison of syntactic representations of two types of syntactic structures: embedded questions and a simple declarative sentence functioning as a probe assertion. Although syntactically simpler than structures like (6) from the BDAE subtest described above, these two structures are also demanding in terms of processing, due to the extensions in embedded questions. B.R. shows that although difficult, this task is not impossible to complete for an agrammatic aphasic: he comprehended both subject and object embedded *who* questions with 1 PP as well as subject *who* and *which NP* embedded questions with 2 PPs above chance.

In general, B.R. shows above chance comprehension of object and chance or below chance comprehension of subject structures in all types of *wh*-dependencies, except in extended embedded and passivized questions. The statistical analyses confirmed the existence of two different patterns in B.R.’s comprehension of *wh*-dependences, with better comprehension of object extractions in direct, long-distance, non-extended embedded questions and relative clasues, and the opposite pattern in his comprehension of extended embedded and passivized questions. It is plausible then to assume that the mechanisms B.R. used in comprehension of direct, long-distance, embedded questions, and relative clauses are different from those used in his comprehension of extended embedded and passivized questions. Thus, it is not his good comprehension of subject extractions in extended embedded and passivized questions that needs an explanation, but rather his poor comprehension of object extractions in these structures.

7.6.3.1.4 Passivized *who/which NP* questions

Note that B.R. scored 1/5 on the BDAE subtest *Passive Subject-Object Discrimination*. However, this does not explain his pattern of comprehension of subject vs. object passivized *who/which* NP questions. The questions in the *Passive* subtest that were asked to determine comprehension of subjects vs. objects in passive *by*-sentences are not passivized questions. It is possible that something related to the preposition *od* "by" contained in the *by*-phrase in Croatian (e.g., *od koga/ od kojeg,-e,-eg NP*) influenced his comprehension of passivized object questions. The *by*-phrase in Croatian passivized object questions appears in the sentence initial position, while in passivized subject questions it appears at the end of a sentence, just as in declarative passive sentences. B.R.'s comprehension of declarative passive sentences with the *by*-phrase that were tested in the *Introductory session* was 7/10, while his comprehension of the same passive structures only without the *by*-phrase was 3/10. It is possible that B.R. relied on the *by*-phrase in the comprehension tasks involving passive constructions. However, when the *by*-phrase occurs at the beginning of the sentence, as in passivized object questions, it is not an unequivocal sign of passive structures any more and the strategy is not operative. For example, the sentence below contains the same phrase that introduces the passivized object questions *od koga/od kojeg NP*, but it is not passivized.

(7) Od koga/od kojeg lava/ zebra bježi?
from who_{Gen}/from which $lion_{Gen}$/ $zebra_{Nom}$ $run_{3sg.pres.}$
"Who/which lion is the zebra running from?"

Thus, since the strategy cannot be applied to passive structures in which the phrase *od koga/kojeg* is either fronted to the sentence initial position or is left out, B.R.'s comprehension of these structures is at chance.

7.6.3.2 *Who-Which NP* Asymmetries in B.R.'s Comprehension

There were 2 statistically significant differences in B.R.'s comprehension of *who* vs. *which NP* structures: he performed better on subject extracted embedded *who* than *which* questions with 2 PPs ($\chi^2(1) = 8.571$, $p = .0034 < .05$), while the opposite pattern was found in object extracted questions: better comprehension of *which* than *who* embedded questions with 1 PP ($\chi^2(1) = 5.000$, $p = .023 < .05$). However, B.R.'s comprehension of either of the last two types of structures did not reach the above chance level (Table 7-11). His overall comprehension on all *wh*-structures is presented in the table below.

Table 7-6.2: B.R.'s overall comprehension of *wh*-structures (percent correct).

B.R.	*Who*	*Which*	Total
Subject	65%	45.7%	54.6%
Object	65%	68.5%	66.92%
Total	65%	57.14%	60.76%

7.7 Case 7: J.Z.

Tako je, kužiš! "That's right, see?" J.Z.

A 67-year-old male was urgently transferred to the Neurological Clinic due to a sudden weakness of the right limbs and speech disturbances. Neurological examination showed right-side hemiparesis and weak reflexes, as well as paresis of the right hypoglossal and facial nerves. A CT scan revealed ischemic lesion in the area supplied by the left middle cerebral artery (MCA) and diffuse atrophic changes in the same area. The patient, J.Z., was diagnosed with an ischemic stroke and mixed nonfluent aphasia. He participated in this study about 7 years after his stroke.

7.7.1 J.Z.'s Performance on Evaluative Measures

J.Z. achieved only 2/14 on the Digit Span, but he scored much better on the RCPM test: 32/36. His performance on the BDAE subtests was poor, as shown in Table 7-7.1.

Table 7-7.1: J.Z.'s scores on the BDAE subtests.

BDAE Scores	
Word Discrimination (/72)	31
Body-Part Identification (/20)	9
Commands (/15)	9
Complex Ideational Material (/12)	6
Supplementary Language Tests	
Passive Subject-Object Discrimination (/5)	2
Indicative vs. Interrogative (/10)	2
Yes-No Questions (/5)	1
Wh-Questions (/5)	1

J.Z.'s scores on the 4 pre-tests of comprehension are as follows: simple declarative *netko:* 5/10, passive *neki NP:* 5/10, passive no-*by*: 2/10, and passive *by* sentences: 4/10.

7.7.2 J.Z.'s Speech Characteristics

J.Z.'s speech is nonfluent, forced, with distortions of phonemes and syllables, and is maximally reduced. He produces at best short phrases, and even then his articulation is halted and impaired.

1. Distortion of phonemes:

- b > p: *porot* instead of *brod* "ship",
- e > a: *padzeset* instead of *pedeset* "fifty",
- č > c: *ocamcto-**cetrdecet*** instead of *osamsto-**četrdeset*** "eight hundred and forty",
- č is sometimes preserved, and even overused: *čječaka* instead of *dječaka* "boy$_{Gen/Acc}$",
- d > dz: *padzeset pet* instead of *pedeset pet* "fifty five",
- g > k: *kotovo : gotovo* "over",
- adding *k* mostly before the vowel of words beginning with a vowel: *kauto* instead of *auto* "car", *kautokpusa canica* for *autobusna stanica* "bus stop",
- *kopao* instead of *pao* "fall$_{lpt.sg.m.}$",
- adding *t* : *troda* instead of *roda* "stork",
- m > b, n > d: *vre**bed**a* instead of *vre**men**a* "time"; *vrije**be*** instead of *vrije**me*** "time"; ***bore*** instead of *more* "sea",
- s > c: *cutra* instead of *sutra* "tomorrow", *cuđe* instead of *suđe* "dishes", *cati* instead of *sati* "time", *cvaku* instead of *svaku* "every", *cupruk* instead of *suprug* "husband",
- z > dz: *jadzero* instead of *jezero* "lake",
- ž > š: *muž > muš* "husband", *puž > puš* "snail", *ruž > ruš* "lipstick".

2. Distortion of syllables

- *gnj > nj:* and *zd > t: njeto* instead of *gnjezdo* "nest",
- st > t: *stolac> tolac* "chair",
- st > s: *kos* instead of *kost* "bone",
- st > c: *ceca* instead of *cesta* "road",
- ts > c: *hrvacik* instead of *hrvatski* "Croatian".

3. Deletion of syllables

- li > ø: *ko-**li**-ko > koko*,

- *kišpati* instead of *kiša padati* “raining”.

Both semantic and phonemic paraphasias are present in J.Z.’s speech, as well as neologisms.

4. Paraphasias

- *Bambi* instead of *lane* “fawn”,
- *kuka* “hook”instead of *ruka* > “arm”,
- *čuka* “bump” instead of *ruka* “arm”,
- *ruka* “arm” instead of *šaka* “hand”.

5. Neologisms:

- *trubičasta* instead of *ljubičasta* “purple”.

This neologism is semantically interesting, consisting of a semantically incorrect stem, *trub-a*, which means “trumpet”, while the remaining part of the adjective is correctly derived.

6. Fillers:

- *Tako je, kužiš*! “That’s right, see?” – J.Z. uses it when he is happy,
- [a 3 -syllable-profanity], *kužiš*! - J.Z. uses it when he is unhappy.

7. Omissions

Future I Tense. Due to omission of the auxiliary (Aux) verb *ću* in the simple future tense, consisting of the Aux and infinitive (e.g., *Sutra ću raditi* “I’ll work tomorrow”), J.Z. produces a truncated sentence with infinitive: *cutra raditi.* Omission of the auxiliary clitic in this verb form results in lack of information on the finitness and time reference, because the main verb takes the form of infinitive in the periphrastic form of future I tense in Croatian.

8. Individual strategies

J.Z. tends to rely on different strategies in order to facilitate speech production and achieve communication. For example, he has no problem saying numbers 1-10, due to relying on rhyming: *jedan-tjedan* “one-week”, *osam-tko sam?* “eight – who am I?”, etc. Without rhyming, he cannot complete the task.

He also resorts to humor. For instance, when the experimenter asked J.Z. “*Kako ćete me pitati kakvo je vrijeme vani*?” (“How would you ask me what the weather is outside?”), instead of making a direct *wh*-question, he responded: “*Ludo!”* “Crazy!” The joke he made implies the time we live in, rather than weather, since the Croatian word *vrijeme* refers to both.

However, it also indicates that he probably did not understand what these two adjoined questions meant, and chose to answer the latter.

7.7.3 J.Z.'s Performance on Experimental Measures

J.Z. comprehended 40.7% of all *wh*-dependencies tested in 4 experiments. He achieved above chance comprehension on only 5 out of 30 structures. Table 7-7.2 shows that percentages on his comprehension of object structures are higher than those on subject structures. Statistical analysis has further shown that, while there was only 1 statistically significant *who-which NP* difference, indicating better comprehension of *who* than *which NP* embedded questions ($\chi^2(1) = 7.500$, $p = .0062 < .05$), there were 8 statistically significant subject-object differences, with 6 of them indicating J.Z.'s better comprehension of the object extractions. The objects-better pattern was found in his comprehension of the following *wh*-structures: direct *who* questions ($\chi^2(1) = 5.051$, $p = .024 < .05$), long distance *who* questions ($\chi^2(1)=4.286$, $p = .0384 < .05$), embedded *who* questions ($\chi^2(1) = 12.800$, $p = .0003 < .05$), direct *which NP* questions ($\chi^2(1) = 9.899$, $p < .0017 < .05$), long-distance-*za which NP* questions ($\chi^2(1) = 4.286$, $p = .0384 < .05$) and relative clauses ($\chi^2(1) = 5.051$, $p = .0246 < .05$).

It is interesting that, like B.R., the cases of J.Z.'s better comprehension of object extractions does not include extended embedded and passivized questions – when there are statistically significant subject-object differences in his comprehension of these structures, they indicate better comprehension of subject extractions. More specifically, unlike B.R., J.Z. comprehended all extended embedded questions at chance. Like B.R., J.Z. showed better comprehension of subject than object extractions in passivized *who* questions ($\chi^2(1) = 5.495$, $p = .019 < .05$) and passivized *which NP* questions ($\chi^2(1) = 7.200$, $p = .0073 < .05$). Thus, it is possible that J.Z. relies on the same comprehension strategy as B.R., which is based on prediction of thematic roles.

Table 7-7.2: J.Z.'s overall comprehension of *wh*-structures (percent correct).

J.Z.	*Who*	*Which*	Total
Subject	35%	32.85%	33.84%
Object	50%	45.71%	47.69%
Total	42.5%	39.28%	40.76%

7.8 Case 8: K.S.

Nema problema. "No problem." K.S.

K.S., a 65-year-old man with a history of hypertension and a stroke that he had suffered 6 years earlier, was hospitalized due to a sudden worsening of weakness in the right limbs and problems in speech and comprehension. A CT scan revealed a new ischemic lesion in the area supplied by the left middle cerebral artery (MCA). Ultrasound examinations showed bilateral plaques in carotid bifurcations and at the origin of both internal carotid arteries, but without significant stenosis. Central lesion of the facial nerve caused the right-side facial paresis. He was diagnosed with mixed fluent aphasia, dyslexia, agraphia, and acalculia.

7.8.1 K.S.'s Performance on Evaluative Measures

K.S. achieved 1/14 on the Digit Span, and 14/34 on the RCPM. His poor results on the RCPM are distinctly worse than the scores of other aphasics, which are in the range of 22-34. The low RCPM scores indicate difficulty with complex visual materials and suggest the possibility that visually parsing and interpreting the scenes of enactment task may have been too difficult for K.S., which in turn might have affected his comprehension scores. His results on the BDAE subtests are also poor, as shown in Table 7-8.1.

Table 7-8.1.K.S.'s scores on the BDAE subtests.

BDAE Scores	
Word Discrimination (/72)	32
Body-Part Identification (/20)	5
Commands (/15)	3
Complex Ideational Material (/12)	1
Supplementary Language Tests	
Passive Subject-Object Discrimination (/5)	2
Indicative vs. Interrogative (/10)	0
Yes-No Questions (/5)	1
Wh-Questions (/5)	2

K.S.'s scores on the 4 pre-tests of comprehension are as follows: simple declarative *netko:* 2/10, passive *neki NP:* 7/10, passive no-*by*: 4/10, and passive *by* sentences: 6/10.

7.8.2 K.S.'s Speech Characteristics

The most prominent characteristic of K.S.'s speech is his awareness of errors he makes and an effort to correct them. Although K.S. produces continuous speech, it consists of circumlocutions, fillers, phonemic and semantic paraphasias as well as neologisms. Very often it is possible to recognize only a few words in the stream of his speech. Self-corrections usually consist of a few trials, leading to successful production of a word. K.S. is more anomic than any of the other 7 aphasics in this study. Examples of his speech errors are listed below.

*1. **Closing of vowels***:

- a > o: ***lo**-va* instead of ***la**-va* "lion$_{Gen / Acc}$"; *zebr-**o*** instead of *zebr-**a*** "zebra" for *zdrijebe,*
- e > o: *sljodi* instead of: *slijedi* or colloquial *sljedi* "follow",
- i > o: *žorafa* instead of *žirafa* "giraffe".

Notice that closing of the vowels *a, e, i* occurs in the first syllable, with the exception of *zebro.* Since there are no reasons for closing the vowel at the end of the word—it would not make articulation easier—perhaps the reason for incorrectly choosing *o* instead of *a* in this particular case is determined by his wrong choice of the noun (*zebra*$_f$ "zebra" was chosen instead of *ždrijebe*$_n$ "foal"), correct choice of the noun gender (neuter), but wrong choice of the noun ending (*-o* as in *nebo*$_n$ "sky" instead of *-e* as in *ždrijebe*$_n$). In other words, he picked a wrong ending (*-o* instead of *-e*) from the correct paradigm (neuter nouns) and combined it with the wrong noun (*zebra* instead of *ždrijebe*). Thus, although making an error in choosing the word *zebra* instead of *ždrijebe,* he correctly chose the type of ending required by the target word, but among the several types of endings for neuter he picked the one that is wrong for the target word (*-o*).

*2. **Distortions of phonemes***

- n > nj *lanje* instead of *lane* "fawn",
- s > ø *leon* instead of *slon* "elephant",
- ž > š; r > v: *kviš* instead of *križ* "cross".

*3. **Paraphasias***

- *pas* "dog" instead of *sat* "watch",
- *baba* "granny" instead of *žaba* "frog",
- *loncem* "pot$_{Instr}$" instead of *novcem* "money$_{Instr}$",
- *mačke* "cat$_{Gen}$" instead of *majke* "mother$_{Gen}$",

- *drvo* “tree” instead of *stablo* “trunk” (whole for a part),
- *u tajnoj sobi* “in a secret room” instead of *u dnevnoj sobi* “in the living room”,
- *brisač* “whiper” instead of *brijač* “barber”,
- *vol* “ox” instead of *lav* “lion”,
- *mrkva* “carrot” instead of *mokra* “wet”,
- *rosonog* instead of *nosorog* “rhino”,
- *doveni konj* instead of *vodeni konj* “hippo”.

4. Neologisms

- *uvruljena* instead of *lovljena* “chased”,
- *sas* instead of *pas* “dog”,
- *divrag* instead of *tigar* “tiger”,
- *severaga* instead of *zebra* “zebra”,
- *cućep* instead of *cvijet* “flower”,
- *puska ladla* instead of *pustinjska deva* “camel”,
- *durnuta* instead of *gurnuta* “pushed”.

5. Circumlocutions

- *bos džungle* “boss of jungle (instead of *kralj džungle* “the king of jungle”) for *lav* “lion”.

6. Grammar

- Past tense > present: *sljubi* > *sljodi* > *sljedi*$_{3sg.pres}$ instead of *slijedio je* “followed$_{3sg.past}$”,
- Aspect: infinite > finite: *lovljena* “chased” > *uvruljena* (nonword).

By substituting the morpheme *lov-* by *vru-*, K.S. produced a nonword: *vruljena.* Interestingly, this nonword has the form of the past participle. In addition, since he attached the prefix *–u* to it, its aspect has changed from imperfective to perfective. These two examples show not only K.S.’s difficulty with the lexical aspect of words, but also with the verb category, in particular with regard to tense and aspect.

7. Fillers

- *Može biti* “It is possible”,
- *To štima* “That's all right”,
- *Bravo!* “Great!”,
- *U tom smislu* “In that sense”,
- *Kako bi' to rek'o*? “How would I put it?”.

7.8.3 K.S.'s Performance on Experimental Measures

K.S. comprehended only 33.8% of all *wh*-dependencies tested in this study, achieving above chance comprehension only in 1 of the 30 types of structures – subject embedded *which NP* questions. There were 2 statistically significant subject-object differences in K.S.'s comprehension, indicating better comprehension of subject extractions: in long-distance *which NP* questions with *za* ($\chi^2(1) = 4.286$, $p = .0384 < .05$) and in embedded *which NP* questions ($\chi^2(1) = 7.500$ $p = .0062 < .05$). There were no significant differences in his comprehension of *who-which NP* structures. The percentage of his comprehension of *wh*-dependencies is summarized in the table below.

Table 7-8.2 K.S.'s overall comprehension of *wh*-structures (percent correct).

K.S.	*Who*	*Which*	Total
Subject	38.3%	38.57%	38.46%
Object	28.3%	30%	29.23%
Total	33.3%	34.2%	33.84%

7.9 Summary of Evaluative and Experimental Measures

7.9.1 Evaluative Measures

The results of each aphasic's performance on the Digit Span, RCPM, BDAE and Supplementary subtests, and introductory evaluative pre-tests are summarized in Table 7-9.

7.9.2 Experimental Measures

Within-case analyses reveal that the Croatian Broca's aphasics showed that their overall comprehension of *wh*-dependencies with subject extractions is equal or close to equal to their comprehension of object extractions in most conditions. Only 21 statistically significant subject-object difference and 4 statistically significant *who-which NP* differences were found in all patients across all conditions. The raw scores are presented in Tables 7-10 and 7-11 below.

Table 7-9: Summary of aphasic patients' performance on the evaluative measures.

Tests	ST	MN	PJ	AD	TP	BR	JZ	KS
RCPM Max score: 36	34	33	31	27	22	25	32	14
DS Max score: 14	8	2	4	2	5	1	2	1
BDAE and Supplementary tests								
Word Discrimination Max score: 72	64	66	64	71	62	45.5	31	32
Body-Part Identification Max score: 20	20	19	19	20	18	16	9	5
Commands Max score: 15	15	15	14	12	9	6	9	3
Complex Ideational Material Max score: 12	10	11	8	10	9	10	6	1
Passive Subject-Object Discrimination Max score: 5	4	5	5	4	4	1	2	2
Indicative vs. Interrogative Max score: 10	10	10	10	8	10	4	2	0
Yes-No Questions Max score: 5	3	5	5	3	2	1	1	1
Wh-Questions Max score: 5	4	5	5	4	2	2	1	2
Pre-tests								
Simple declarative *netko* Max score: 10	10	9	10	10	7	8	5	2
Passive *neki NP* Max score: 10	10	7	10	10	7	9	5	7
Passive no-by Max score: 10	10	10	10	10	6	3	2	4
Passive-by Max score: 10	10	10	10	10	9	7	4	6

Table 7-10 presents each case in a column, and each condition in a row. The results are divided into three groups of structures, depending on the type of *wh*-word they contain: *tko* "who", *koji NP* "which NP" and *koji* "which". Each of these groups consists of the raw scores for subject and object extractions within each type of *wh*-dependencies (rows) for each participant (column). For example, J.Z. achieved a score of 2 on direct *who* subject, and 7 on direct *who* object questions. In Table 7-10, scores above the chance level are given in bold, those at chance are in italics, while the below chance scores are underlined.

Table 7.10: Comprehension of Different Structures with Subject (S) vs. Object (O) Extractions.

S vs. O	S.T.	M.N.	P.J.	A.D.	T.P.	B.R.	J.Z.	K.S.
Tko	S O	S O	S O	S O	S O	S O	S O	S O
DQ	**10 10**	**10 10**	**9 9**	**10 10**	**10 10**	*4* **9** $p < .05$	*2* **7** $p < .05$	*6 2*
LD	**5 5**	**5 5**	**5 4**	**4 5**	**4 4**	*0* **5** $p < .05$	*0 3* $p < .05$	*2 0*
LD *za*	**5 5**	**5 5**	**4 5**	**5 4**	*2* **4**	**4 4**	*0 1*	*1 0*
EQ	**10 8**	**10 10**	**10 9**	**10 9**	*5* **10** $p < .05$	*4* **9** $p < .05$	*1* **9** $p < .05$	*5 2*
EQ1PP	**9 8**	*5* **8**	*5* **8**	*5 6*	*4 5*	**8** <u>0</u> $p < .05$	*5 5*	*4 4*
EQ2PP	**10 8**	*5* **9**	*7* **9**	*5 6*	*7 5*	**10 8**	*7 4*	*4 4*
PQ	**10 9**	**9 9**	*5 5*	**10 10**	**8 8**	**9** *4* $p < .05$	*6 1* $p < .05$	*1 5*
Koji NP	S O	S O	S O	S O	S O	S O	S O	S O
DQ	**9 10**	**10 8**	**9 7**	**8 9**	**8 8**	*1* **7** $p < .05$	1 **8** $p < .05$	*4 1*
LD	**4 5**	**5 5**	**5 4**	**4 4**	**4 5**	*1* **5** $p < .05$	*0* 2	2 *0*

LD *za*	**5 5**	**5 5**	**5 4**	**5 5**	**4 5**	*1* **4**	*0 3* $p < .05$	*3 0* $P < .05$
EQ	**10 10**	**10 10**	**9 10**	**9 10**	**7 8**	2 **8** $p < .05$	1 *3*	**7** 1 $p < .05$
EQ1PP	**9 8**	*5 7*	*5 6*	*7 6*	*4 4*	**9** *6*	*6 3*	*3 6*
EQ2PP	*7* **9**	**8** *6*	*5* **9**	*5 7*	*3 5*	*4 6*	*5 4*	1 *5*
PQ	**10 10**	**9 10**	**7 9**	**8** *6*	**8 8**	**10** 2 $p < .05$	**8** *2* $p < .05$	*1 5*
Koji	S O	S O	S O	S O	S O	S O	S O	S O
RC	**9 9**	**9 9**	**9 7**	**9 9**	**8 8**	*4* **10** $p < .05$	2 **7** $p < .05$	*6 3*

Table 7-11: Comprehension of *Who* (T) vs. *Which NP* (K) dependencies by 8 aphasics.

T vs. K	S.T.	M.N.	P.J.	A.D.	T.P.	B.R.	J.Z.	K.S
Subject	**T K**	**T K**	**T K**	**T K**	**T K**	**T K**	**T K**	**T K**
DQ	**10 9**	**10 10**	**9 9**	**10 8**	**10 8**	*4 1*	*2 1*	*6 4*
EQ	**10 10**	**10 10**	**10 9**	**10 9**	5 7	4 *2*	*1 1*	*5* **7**
LD	**5 5**	**5 5**	**5 5**	**4 4**	**4 4**	*0 1*	*0 0*	*2 2*
LD *za*	**5 5**	**5 5**	**4 5**	**5 5**	*2* **4**	**4** 1	*0 0*	*1 3*
PQ	**10 10**	**9 9**	*5* **7**	**10 8**	**8 8**	**9 10**	*6* **8**	*1 1*
EQ1PP	**9 9**	*5 5*	*5 5*	*5 7*	4 4	**8 9**	*5 6*	*4 3*
EQ2PP	**10** 7	5 **8**	*7 5*	*5 5*	*7 3*	**10** 4 $p < .05$	*7 5*	*4* 1
Object	**T K**	**T K**	**T K**	**T K**	**T K**	**T K**	**T K**	**T K**
DQ	**10 10**	**10 8**	**9 7**	**10 9**	**10 8**	**9 7**	**7 8**	*2 1*
EQ	**8 10**	**10 10**	**9 10**	**9 10**	**10 8**	**9 8**	**9** *3* $p <.05$	*2 1*
LD	**5 5**	**5 5**	**4 4**	**5 4**	**4 5**	**5 5**	*3* 2	*0 0*

LD *za*	**5 5**	**5 5**	**5 4**	**4 5**	**4 5**	**4 4**	*1 3*	*0 0*
PQ	**9 10**	**9 10**	*5* **9**	**10 6** p <.05	**8 8**	*4 2*	*1 2*	*5 5*
EQ1PP	**8 8**	8 *7*	**8** *6*	*6 6*	*5 4*	0 *6* p < .05	*5 3*	*4 6*
EQ2PP	**8 9**	**9** *6*	**9 9**	*6 7*	*5 5*	**8** *6*	*4 4*	*4 5*

In Table 7-11, the results are presented from a different perspective. Here, the results are divided into 2 groups: Subject and Object Extractions. Within each of these groups the raw scores for *who* and *which NP* questions on each type of *wh*-dependencies are presented together for each participant. For example, S.T. had a score of 10 on *who* and 9 on *which NP* direct questions. Relative clauses do not appear in the table as they involve only one type of *wh*-phrase. As in Table 7-10, here too the scores above chance are given in bold, those at chance are in italics, while the below-chance scores are underlined.

Of 8 patients, 5 were agrammatic aphasics, with either Broca's aphasia (M.N., P.J.) or with a mixed nonfluent aphasia (T.P., B.R. and J.Z.). Two of these patients, M.N. and P.J. did not display any statistically significant asymmetries. However, B.R. showed 10 subject-object asymmetries and 2 *who-which NP* asymmetries, J.Z. showed 8 and T.P. 1 statistically significant subject-object asymmetry. There was also 1 *who-which NP* asymmetry in J.Z. Participant K.S., who had a mixed fluent aphasia, exhibited chance comprehension of most structures. He displayed only 2 statistically significant subject-object differences.

The remaining two patients, A.D. and S.T., were not agrammatic. A.D. is a non-agrammatic Broca's aphasic who displayed a comprehension pattern similar to that found in agrammatic Broca's patients, with the exception of 1 *who-which NP* asymmetry found in her comprehension of passivized questions. Finally, S.T. is an anomic aphasic speaker who comprehended *wh*-dependencies at ceiling (92.6%). The only exception was the subject embedded *koji NP* questions with 2 PPs, which she comprehended at chance. Since S.T.'s scores are at ceiling and K.S.'s at floor, they will not be much discussed in the rest of the book. I will instead focus on the results from the three Broca's patients and three cases of mixed nonfluent aphasia (Chapter 8).

Thus, from the experimental results for Broca's aphasics, agrammatic and non-agrammatic, we can conclude that the Croatian data do not fit the pattern reported for English-speaking Broca's aphasics. It is interesting to find no statistically significant differences in comprehension of subject vs. object *who/which NP* dependencies among Broca's aphasics and to find most of significant differences in patients with mixed nonfluent aphasia. The data are summarized in Table 7-12 below.

Table 7-12. Comparison to chance level of scores on all structures for each case study: > "above chance", = "at chance", < "below chance"; * represents statistically significant subject-object differences, and ^ represents statistically significant *who-which* differences.

		DQ		EQ		LD		LD-za		EQ1PP		EQ2PP		RC	PQ	
		who	whi	who	whi	who	whi	who	whi	who	whi	who	whi	whi	who	whi
ST	S	>	>	>	>	>	>	>	>	>	>	>	=	>	>	>
	O	>	>	>	>	>	>	>	>	>	>	>	>	>	>	>
MN	S	>	>	>	>	>	>	>	>	=	=	=	>	>	>	>
	O	>	>	>	>	>	>	>	>	>	=	>	=	>	>	>
AD	S	>	>	>	>	>	>	>	>	=	=	=	=	>	>	>
	O	>	>	>	>	>	>	>	>	=	=	=	=	>	>^	>^
PJ	S	>	>	>	>	>	>	>	>	=	=	=	=	>	=	>
	O	>	>	>	>	>	>	>	>	>	=	>	>	>	=	>
TP	S	>	>	=*	>	>	>	=	>	=	=	=	=	>	>	>
	O	>	>	>*	>	>	>	>	>	=	=	=	=	>	>	>
JZ	S	=*	=*	=*	=	=*	=	=	=*	=	=	=	=	=*	=*	>*
	O	>*	>*	>*^	=^	=*	=	=	=*	=	=	=	=	>*	=*	=*
BR	S	=*	=*	=*	=*	=*	=*	>	=	>*	>	>^	=^	=*	>*	>*
	O	>*	>*	>*	>*	>*	>*	>	>	<*^	=^	>	=	>*	=*	=*
KS	S	=	=	=	>*	=	=	=	=*	=	=	=	<	=	=	=
	O	=	=	=	=*	=	=	=	=*	=	=	=	=	=	=	=

It appears then that overall comprehension of subject vs. object *who/which NP* dependencies was equal or close to equal in Broca's aphasics. Chance performance on both subject and object *wh*-dependencies is the next prevalent pattern, which is followed by the pattern of better comprehension of *wh*-dependencies with object extractions, which was found in cases with mixed nonfluent aphasia. Thus, the data do not fit the pattern reported for English-speaking Broca's aphasics. Although mixed nonfluent aphasia resembles Broca's aphasia, these patients' comprehension is in general more impaired than Broca's aphasics' comprehension. The Croatian data further support this observation.

7.10 The Control Subjects

Three healthy native speakers of Croatian, A.K., O.P., and C.H., two female and one male, age range 64-67 (mean age: 65.3), participated as control subjects in the study. Their results on the RCPM[1] were: AK 35/36, O.P. 35/36, and C.H. 36/36. The results of all experiments with the Croatian control speakers are presented in Table 7-13 below. All control subjects achieved above chance comprehension of all tested structures, with the exception of O.P., who achieved 70% correct comprehension of embedded subject *which NP* questions with 1 PP, which is chance level performance.

Chance comprehension on some extended embedded *wh*-questions was also found in a study with healthy elderly native speakers of Spanish (Kljajevic & Fratini, 2011). The study tested comprehension of direct questions, embedded questions with 1 and 2 PPs, and relative clauses in elderly and young control participants in 3 experiments. The stimuli from Experiment 3 in the present study were translated into and adapted to Spanish, and used to test auditory comprehension of subject and object *who* ("quién") and *which NP* ("qué") embedded questions with 1 and 2 extensions in 11 neurologically intact elderly native speakers of Spanish. The healthy elderly participants, who were within the age range 60 and 85, had a score of 26 or better on the Montreal Cognitive Assessment (MoCA) test, which indicates that their cognitive status was normal. In addition, 10 elderly persons whose MoCA scores were less than 26, which indicates a Mild Cognitive Impairment, and 18 young individuals with the MoCA score of 26 or better, were also tested on the same structures. While the

[1] Since the control subjects were tested only on the Digit Span forward but not backward, like the aphasic participants, the control group's Digit Span results are not reported here.

Table 7-13. Control subjects' performance on experimental measures.

S vs. O	A.K.		O.P.		C.H.	
Tko						
DQ	10	10	10	10	10	10
LD	5	5	5	4	5	5
LD *za*	5	5	5	5	4	5
EQ	10	10	10	10	10	10
EQ1PP	10	9	8	8	10	10
EQ2PP	8	10	8	9	10	9
PQ	10	10	10	9	9	8
Koji NP						
DQ	10	10	9	8	10	10
LD	5	5	5	5	5	5
LD *za*	5	5	5	5	5	5
EQ	10	9	10	10	10	10
EQ1PP	10	10	7	9	10	10
EQ2PP	10	8	9	8	8	9
PQ	9	10	8	9	10	10
Koji						
RC	10	9	9	10	10	10

elderly persons with low MoCA scores performed at chance level on all types of extended embedded questions, and young controls comprehended all of them above chance, the healthy elderly with MoCA score of 26 and better comprehended embedded subject and object *who* questions with 1 PP as well as their embedded object *who* questions with 2 PPs at chance. Note that this group's comprehension of other types of embedded questions (i.e., subject *which NP* questions), subject and object direct *who* and *which NP* questions as well as subject and object relative clauses was above chance. Thus, the evidence from Spanish with healthy elderly inividuals indicates that embedded questions with 1 and 2 PPs are in general difficult to process for the elderly, even though grammatical knowledge is intact in this population – which indicates a processing limitation.

CHAPTER EIGHT

GENERAL DISCUSSION

8.1 The Main Findings of the Study

The experimental results presented in Chapter 7 reveal that Croatian Broca's aphasics who participated in this study do not follow the pattern of comprehension of *wh*-questions that has been reported for English-speaking Broca's aphasics. In English, the pattern of asymmetric comprehension of *who* vs. *which NP* questions consists of good comprehension of both subject and object *who* questions as well as subject *which NP* questions, and poor comprehension of object *which NP* questions (Hickok & Avrutin, 1996). This pattern was not found in Croatian Broca's aphasics (M.N., P.J. and A.D.), or in cases with mixed aphasia, nonfluent (T.P., B.R. and J.Z.) or fluent (K.S.). Some asymmetry was found in the Croatian patients with mixed aphasia, but it does not match the pattern found in English aphasic patients.

8.1.1 Overall Performance of All Aphasics

Looking at the performance of all eight Croatian aphasics across all conditions we find 21 subject-object asymmetry and 4 *who-which NP* statistically significant differences. In 14/21 subject-object asymmetries, comprehension of *wh*-dependencies with extraction from object position was better than comprehension of structures with extraction from subject position, while only in 7/21 subject-object asymmetries the pattern was opposite, with better comprehension of the subject extractions. Only 4 statistically significant *who-which NP* differences were found across all conditions in all 8 patients, and one of these asymmetries was between the scores that were at chance and below chance levels of comprehension. Now I turn to Croatian Broca's and cases of mixed nonfluent aphasia in order to establish the dominant pattern in their comprehension of subject vs. object *who/which NP* dependencies.

8.1.2 Broca's Aphasics and Cases with Mixed Nonfluent Aphasia

Croatian Broca's aphasics A.D., M.N. and P.J. displayed no asymmetries in comprehension of subject vs. object *who/which NP* dependencies. Patients with mixed nonfluent aphasia B.R. and J.Z. showed a pattern of better comprehension of structures with extraction from object position than structures with extraction from subject position, except for T.P. who followed this pattern only in comprehension of embedded *who* questions and whose comprehension resembled more the pattern of Broca's aphasics, which is lack of asymmetry. Patient K.S., whose language deficit matched mixed fluent aphasia, exhibited chance-level comprehension, and showed 2 subject-object *who/which NP* asymmetries, which ran in the direction opposite to the pattern found in the cases of mixed nonfluent aphasia.

8.1.2.1 Broca's Aphasics: A.D., M.N. and P.J.

A.D., M.N. and P.J. differ in several respects. First, while A.D. is not agrammatic, M.N. and P.J. are agrammatic, displaying similar features in speech output (see Chapter 7, sections 7.2 and 7.3). Second, while A.D. and M.N. had one cerebral accident, P.J. had two strokes. Both A.D. and P.J. are right-handed, while M.N. is ambidextrous. Since ambidextrous persons are likely to have a more bilateral representation of language, they have better recovery prognosis (Ferro & Madureira, 2002). Further, the type and size of lesion differ in these three patients, indicating the possibility of different recovery prognosis: A.D.'s lesion is cortical, in M.N. it is cortico-subcortical, while P.J.'s lesion is subcortical. A.D. had stenosis at the origin of the left ICA. In addition to the ischemic lesion, atherosclerotic changes found in this patient could have also contributed to her language disturbances, given that such systemic disorders usually affect many aspects of cognition. M.N. had a temporo-parietal cortico-subcortical ischemic lesion of size 4 x 3 x 4 cm. In addition to this, he had two chronic lacunar lesions in the left basal ganglia, in the left putamen and in the left caudate nuclei. P.J. had two strokes, the first of which left a big lesion in the left basal ganglia, more specifically in the internal capsule, spreading to the anterior horn of the lateral ventricle. The second stroke left a lesion smaller than the first one (around 2 cm) subcortically, in the left lenticular nucleus, expanding to the anterior horn of the left lateral ventricle. In addition, P.J. has been diagnosed with Moya-Moya, a disease that is expected to cause additional changes in the brain vasculature, causing in turn further changes in cognition and behaviour. Thus, it seems that the differences with regard to number, location, and size of lesions in these three patients were not a differentiating factor in their comprehension of subject and object extractions in *wh*-dependencies, given that they all showed the same pattern, that is *no asymmetry*.

8.1.2.2 Cases of Mixed Nonfluent Aphasia: T.P., B.R. and J.Z.

Patients T.P., B.R. and J.Z. have been diagnosed with mixed non-fluent aphasia. They are all agrammatic, but they display different degrees of disturbances of grammatical relations in speech production and comprehension. What these three patients have in common is that none of them had more than one stroke. Also, all three patients have residual right-side hemiparesis, as well as residual right-side facial paresis. In addition to damage to the facial nerve, J.Z. and B.R. had the hypoglossal nerve affected, which additionally has burdened their articulation. However, T.P., B.R. and J.Z. differ with regard to the type of stroke they had, and location of lesion. While T.P. and J.Z. had an ischemic stroke, B.R. had an intracerebral hemorrhage. Ischemia and hemorrhage are "different mechanisms of brain damage" in stroke, with different preferences for anatomic brain loci (Caplan, 2000) and different prognosis for recovery.

> After a hemorrhagic stroke, the residual lesion is much smaller than the initial hematoma; it usually spares the cortex and it is of smaller size than an infarct causing aphasia of similar acute severity. Aphasia secondary to intracerebral hemorrhage usually recovers better than that due to infarcts of similar size (Ferro & Madureira, 2002, p. 152).

B.R. had a big subcortical hematoma in the left basal ganglia spreading to the left lateral ventricle. T.P. had a 3 x 2 cm occlusive lesion at the origin of ICA, extending cortico-subcortically, stenosis of the left ICA for 40%, asymmetric circulation of the Willis circle with zero circulation in the left external carotid artery, narrower left Sylvian fissure and the left temporo-parietal sulci. J.Z.'s lesion is cortical, at the origin of the left MCA. Thus, these three patients' distribution of lesions is also uneven, running subcortically, cortico-subcortically, and cortically.

These three patients exhibited different patterns in comprehension of *wh*-dependencies. T.P., whose lesion site is similar to A.D.'s, showed only 1 asymmetry across all conditions, with the rest of his scores patterning with those of Broca's aphasics and indicating lack of subject-object *who/which NP* asymmetry in comprehension. However, despite the fact that different stroke mechanisms (ischemia vs. hemorrhage) caused lesions that also differed in their distribution (cortical vs. subcortical) in J.Z. and B.R., these two patients' scores patterned together on most conditions. One prominent pattern in their comprehension of *wh*-dependencies is better comprehension of structures with extraction from object position compared to structures with extraction from subject position. Interestingly, the opposite pattern prevailed in these patients' comprehension of passivized and extended embedded questions (see Section 8.2).

8.1.3 A Case of Mixed Fluent Aphasia: K.S.

K.S. is the only case of fluent mixed aphasia. Like P.J., he had two strokes, the first of which resulted in Broca's aphasia (no data available on the lesion site). The second stroke affected the left MCA at the origin, resulting in a mixed fluent aphasia. His performance on evaluative measures shows signs of decline in areas other than language (recall his low scores on the Digit Span and RCPM). This patient showed a predominant pattern of chance performance and minimal asymmetry, consisting of 2 statistically significant subject-object differences reflecting better comprehension of subject than object *wh*-dependencies.

8.1.4 Summary of the Main Findings

The results clearly show that Croatian Broca's aphasics as well as cases with nonfluent and fluent mixed aphasia do not follow the pattern of comprehension of *wh*-dependencies found in English speaking Broca's aphasics. Three comprehension patterns were discerned: equal or close to equal comprehension of subject vs. object *who-which NP* dependencies (Broca's aphasics), better comprehension of object compared to subject extractions (mixed nonfluent aphasics) and better comprehension of subject compared to object extractions (mixed nonfluent aphasics).

It appears that different lesion sites in the Croatian aphasics (for example, at the origin of ICA, at the origin of MCA, at the areas supplied by the branches of MCA, in the basal ganglia, the area supplied by PCA) are associated with the same pattern(s) of comprehension of *wh*-dependencies. In other words, based on the Croatian data we cannot discern a specific lesion site associated with a distinct pattern of comprehension of *wh*-dependencies.

8.2 Computing *Wh*-Dependencies

Broca's aphasics, M.N., P.J. and A.D., showed above chance comprehension of both subject and object structures formed by *who* and *which NP* in the following conditions: direct, long distance questions with- and without the preposition *za*, and embedded questions. Since their comprehension of passivized and extended embedded questions is poorer, with chance comprehension on some of these structures, I now turn to these two conditions in order to determine their syntactic complexity and processing demands.

8.2.1 Passivized Questions

All 4 types of passivized questions tested in this study contain the *by*-phrase. Comprehension of the *by*-phrase was pre-tested on structures like (1) that involve NP-movement only, and not *wh*-movement.

(1) a. *e* was followed the giraffe by the camel
b. The giraffe$_i$ was followed t_i by the camel

The sentence shown in (1) above is formed by movement of the underlying object *the giraffe* from the D-structure, shown in (1a), to subject position in S-structure, shown in (1b).

With passive questions, there are two *wh*-phrases that may be questioned: the matrix subject (see (2)), and the object of the preposition *by*, as shown in (3). In (2b) *which giraffe* raises from the D-structure object position to the subject position, leaving a co-indexed trace behind with which it forms an A-chain. It then undergoes *wh*-movement, forming another chain, this time an A'-chain (2c).

Subject passivized question
(2) a. *e* was followed which giraffe by the camel
b. which giraffe$_i$ was followed t_i by the camel - NP-movement
c. which giraffe$_j$ t_j was followed by the camel - *Wh*-movement

In (3) it is the object of the preposition *by* that undergoes NP-movement (3b) and *wh*-movement (3c).

Object passivized question

(3) a. the giraffe was followed by which camel

b. which camel$_i$ was the giraffe followed by t_i - NP-movement

c. which camel$_j$ t_j was the giraffe followed by - *Wh*-movement

Passivized questions in Croatian undergo similar process of *wh*-movement preceded by NP-movement. Note, however, that there is a structural difference between English and Croatian passivized object questions. In English, passivized object questions are formed by movement from a PP, like in (4).

(4) Who$_i$ /which camel$_i$ was the giraffe followed [$_{PP}$ by t$_i$]?

In Croatian, the whole PP moves to the front, leaving no overt phrasal element behind, as shown in (5).

(5) [$_{PP}$ Od koga$_i$]/[$_{PP}$ od koje deve$_i$] je žirafa slijeđena t$_i$?

by who$_{Gen}$ / by which camel$_{Gen}$ Aux$_{3sg.pres}$ giraffe$_{Nom}$ follow$_{lpt.sg.f.}$

"Who/which camel was the giraffe followed by?"

This difference in passivized object questions suggests that their comprehension is perhaps computationally more demanding in English than in Croatian, because the movement involves extraction out of an extra layer of structure, the PP. Since this does not happen in Croatian, we can expect better comprehension of passivized questions in Croatian than in English aphasics, and approximately the same level of comprehension of subject and object *tko* and *koji NP* passivized questions in Croatian aphasics.

Four Broca's aphasics tested by Thompson et al. (1999) performed mostly at chance level on passivized subject-object *who* and *which NP* questions. For instance, M.D. comprehended all passivized questions at chance, D.L. comprehended only object *who* questions above chance, F.P. only subject *who* questions, and C.H. comprehended only subject *which NP* questions above chance. Given the structural complexity of English passivized questions, the controversial status of *who/which NP* dependencies and inconsistent results across strudies reported in the literature, it is hard to explain Thompson et al.'s data on passivized *who/ which NP* questions. However, the data do indicate that the pattern consisting of good comprehension of subject and object *who* and subject *which NP* questions, and poor comprehension of object *which NP* questions does not generalize to passivized questions. The Croatian data, on the other side, clearly show lack of the subject-object *who/which NP* asymmetric pattern in Broca's aphasics, which is consistent with Croatian Broca's aphasics' overall performance.

8.2.2 Extended Embedded Questions

M.N., P.J. and A.D. exhibited a discrepancy in comprehension of non-extended embedded questions (Experiment 1) and embedded questions with 1 or 2 PPs (Experiment 3). While they comprehended nonextended embedded *who* and *which NP* questions above chance, without regard to the type of extraction (subject or object), their performance on embedded questions with 1 or 2 PPs was less accurate. On these structures P.J. and M.N. performed at chance on both subject and object embedded *which NP* questions with 1 extension, on subject *who* with 1 extension, and subject *who* with 2 extensions. While M.N. performed at chance on object *which NP* embedded questions with 2 extensions, M.N. performed at chance on the subject *which NP* embedded questions with 2 extensions. Surprisingly, A.D. performed at chance level on all types of extended embedded questions. Since the same sentence structure, tested in Experiment 1, is extended by 1 or 2 PPs in sentences in Experiment 3, from the discrepancy in their comprehension of sentences in these two experiments we can conclude that it is not the syntactic complexity of the basic embedded question structure that caused comprehension difficulty with extended embedded questions in these patients. We must, therefore, examine the differences in methodology and computational demands in the two experiments.

Recall that embedded questions without extensions were tested within the act-out paradigm, having a structure such as (6).

(6) Pokaži mi koja žirafa je slijedila zebru.
"Show me which giraffe followed the zebra."

The structure of embedded sentences with extensions, however, is as follows:

(7) Petar zna *tko* je [u utorak] [iz telefonske govornice] doktora zvao.
Peter knows who [on Tuesday] [from a phone booth] called the doctor.
"Peter knows who called the doctor from a phone booth on Tuesday."

As in (6), the structure in (7) requires that certain structural elements be stored and processed in WM while attending to the rest of the sentence.

However, the structure in (7) is computationally more demanding than that in (6), for at least two reasons. First, in addition to an embedded question, it is accompanied by a probe assertion, as in (8), to which the patient must answer "Correct" or "Incorrect".

(8) The doctor called the patient.

Although simple in structure, probe assertions still require full attention, while at the same time the semantic interpretation of the embedded question needs to be stored so that it can be compared with that of the probe assertion. In order to come up with an answer, a patient needs to perform a computationally demanding sequence of tasks. Thus, not only was the tested sentence lengthened by adding 1 or 2 PPs, but the overall processing demand was also increased by applying a verification paradigm with probe assertions. Second, unlike in the act-out task, where the toy animals were left on the table after the action was acted out, there were no visual cues to facilitate memory processes in this paradigm. Therefore, the processing demand in the embedded questions with 1 or 2 PPs was greatly increased. This is reflected in chance-level comprehension of 3 out of 4 types of *which NP* extended embedded questions and 2 out of 4 types of *who* extended embedded questions by M.N. and P.J., as well as in chance-level comprehension of 8 out of 8 types of extended embedded questions by A.D.

However, in spite of the increased load, M.N. and P.J. performed above chance on embedded object *who* questions with 1 and 2 extensions. P.J. achieved above chance on object *koji NP* with 2 extensions as well, while M.N. showed the reverse result, performing above chance with the subject rather than the object questions. Perhaps they relied on the same strategy that patients with mixed nonfluent aphasia used in comprehension of structures on which they showed better comprehension of structures with extraction from object than subject position.

Patient A.D. shows a consistent pattern of chance performance on *who* and *which NP* extended embedded subject and object questions with 1 and 2 extensions. Overall, she performed at chance level on 9 out of 30 types of *wh*-structures, with 8 of them revealing chance comprehension of all extended embedded questions (the ninth one tests passivized object *which NP* questions). Given that A.D. comprehended above chance the remaining 21 types of *wh*-structures, including the non-lengthened embedded questions (Experiment 1), one could argue that her knowledge of syntax may be preserved. That would evoke a processing explanation: chance performance on extended embedded questions results from an inability to attend to the sentence as it unfolds in time while simultaneously building the representations.

The problem can be in syntactic WM, i.e., due to an inability to assign enough processing resources to establishing proper dependency relations between the dislocated element and its trace. The longer the distance between the two, the bigger the processing load. Alternatively, the problem might be an inability to assign enough processing resources necessary for integration of the dislocated constituent and its subcategorizing verb. Clearly, sentences in (9) and (10) impose different processing loads, with the latter example representing the stimuli used in Experiment 3.

(9) Petar zna *koga*$_i$ je$_j$ doktor t_j zvao t_i
Peter know$_{3sg.pres.}$ who$_{Acc}$ AUX$_{3sg.pres.}$ doctor$_{Nom}$ call$_{lpt.sg.m.}$
"Peter knows who the doctor called."

(10) Petar zna koga$_i$ je$_j$ [u utorak]
[iz javne govornice] doktor t_j zvao t_i
Peter know$_{3sg.pres.}$ who$_{Acc}$ AUX$_{3sg.pres.}$ [on Tuesday]
[from phone booth] doctor$_{Nom}$ call$_{lpt.sg.m.}$
"Peter knows who the doctor called on Tuesday afternoon from a phone booth."

Recall that in Croatian inflectional case endings mark the grammatical function of a declined NP. In this case, *koga* is the Accusative of *tko* "who", which indicates that its grammatical function is the direct object of the sentence. A noun in Accusative, which functions as a direct object in a sentence, is usually assigned the thematic role of Patient. Thus, based on the case ending, the parser can predict the grammatical function of the inflected word and a corresponding thematic role. If this is the case, then most of the syntactic representation can be built based on available grammatical information and predictions on thematic roles even before the verb is encountered, which further facilitates comprehension. It is clear, of course, that actual thematic role assignment can take place only after the verb has been encountered.

Also, the verb phrase (VP) in the example above is disjointed by two inserted phrases:

(11) je [PP] [PP] zvao
AUX$_{3sg.pres.}$ [PP] [PP] call$_{lpt.sg.m.}$
"(he) has called"

It is possible that the auxiliary, by agreeing with the verb in number, contributes to parsing by enabling correct predictions on the agreement features of the main verb. Thus, simply by appearing right after the *wh*-constituent, *je* "has" has already brought in some features of *zvao* "called". At this point, however, the whole process is interrupted by the insertion of two phrases modifying the action expressed by the verb, which is still unknown to the parser.

Note also that the *wh*-constituent in *which NP* questions in Experiment 3 is disrupted by the auxiliary *je:*

(12) Petar zna koji je doktor u utorak iz telefonske govornice pacijenta zvao.
Peter knows $which_{Nom}$ $AUX_{3.sg.pres.}$ $doctor_{Nom}$ on Tuesday from a phone booth $patient_{Acc}$ $call_{lpt.sg.m.}$
"Peter knows which doctor called the patient on Tuesday from a phone booth."

The auxiliary clitic *je* carries information that is crucial for the minimal clause formation. For example, the 3rd person singular form *je* indicates that the following element is also in singular (*Koji je pacijent zvao doktora?* "Which patient called the doctor?"), while the 3nd person plural form *su* indicates plural (*Koji su pacjenti zvali doktora*? "Which patients called the doctor?"). Thus, the parser immediately obtains information on the number from the auxiliary verb, instead of waiting to extract this information from the noun suffix. Resolving the potential ambiguity of *koji NP* before the second noun is encountered could speed up or facilitate processing. Note however that the ambiguity with regard to number holds for Nominative, but not for *koji NP* in Accusative, where the case ending unambiguously marks the number at the same time (*$Kojeg_{Acc.sg.}$ je $pacijenta_{Acc.sg.}$ doktor zvao? $Koje_{Acc.pl.}$ je $pacijente_{Acc.pl.}$ doktor zvao?*).

Once the Agent is encountered, thematic predictions on the Accusative form of *tko* serving as a Patient or Theme in a sentence becomes even more likely, to be finally confirmed in the next step, i.e., during the filler-verb integration. Even though it is not possible to assign thematic roles without knowing the meaning of a verb, correctly predicting thematic roles from grammatical functions probably speeds up processing, making unused resources available to other processes in comprehension. As a final step, the *wh*-constituent gets associated with its trace. Thus, there are several structural cues that could "guide" comprehension while parsing extended embedded object questions in Croatian.

Returning to A.D.'s overall performance in light of the discussion on processing resources, it is rather striking to find that she performed at chance level on all types of extended embedded questions, while performing above chance on structures of a higher degree of syntactic complexity, such as long-distance questions. It is certainly the case that long-distance dependencies are also computationally taxing, but at least in the case of A.D., failure to comprehend embedded questions with 1 or 2 extensions at a level better than chance indicates that it is a processing rather than syntactic deficit.

8.3 Syntactic Explanations of the Lack of Asymmetry in Broca's Aphasics Data

The first general claim at which we arrive when we compare the results of this study with the data reported in the literature is that Broca's aphasics, both English and Croatian, do not exhibit a single pattern of comprehension deficit. For that reason, syntactic explanations of the results obtained from English-speaking aphasic patients fail to account for the Croatian data.

8.3.1 *Who* vs. *Which NP*

Since only 1 statistically significant difference was found in comprehension of *tko* vs. *koji NP* questions across all conditions in Broca's aphasics (see Table 7-11), the first question to explore is: *Is there a syntactic difference between* tko *and* koji NP *in Croatian?*

Wh-word-order in Croatian is described in Chapter 3, where it was shown that a *wh*-word has to occupy a sentence- or clause-initial position, and that, provided that this requirement is satisfied, *wh*-words in a sentence can switch between subject and object positions. Similarly, Rudin's (1988) analysis of Serbo-Croatian multiple short-distance *tko* and *što* "what" questions shows that this language does not impose a strict order on *wh*-words that appear in multiple *wh*-questions. Recall from Chapter 4 that the Superiority Condition determined that there was a syntactic difference between *who/what* and *which NP*, since *who* and *what* obey the Superiority Condition, but *which NP* does not.

(13) a. *What$_i$ did who buy t$_i$?
b. Who$_i$ t$_i$ bought what?
(14) a. Which book$_i$ did which girl buy t$_i$?
b. Which girl$_i$ t$_i$ bought which book?

As shown in (13a), *what* has been moved across another *wh*-phrase: *who*. *Who* is now superior (higher up in the tree) to the trace left behind *what,* with which it is not co-indexed. Thus, the sentence in (13a) violates the Superiority Condition and is ungrammatical. On the other hand, (13b) involves no crossing and then is grammatical. However, since the Superiority Condition does not apply to *which NP* phrases, either subject or object *which NP* phrases can move to Spec CP, as shown in (14a-b).

If the Superiority Condition does not exist in Croatian (as also claimed by Rudin, 1988), then there are no syntactic differences between *tko* and *koji* in the *wh*-dependencies examined in this study, which in turn explains the lack of comprehension differences in Broca's aphasic patients.

However, Bošković (1997) claims that in Serbo-Croatian, as in English, D-linked *wh*-words (e.g., *koji NP*) do not obey Superiority requirements. Otherwise, he claims, "SC [Serbo-Croatian] is well behaved with respect to Superiority: It exhibits Superiority effects whenever *wh*-movement takes place" (p. 12). If this is true, and syntactic differences between *tko* and *koji NP* exist, then the question is: *How to explain the lack of asymmetry in Croatian Broca's aphasics' comprehension of* who *vs.* which NP *dependencies?*

Returning to the proposed explanations of the syntactic comprehension deficit in Broca's aphasia presented in Chapter 4, an attempt to explain the lack of asymmetry in comprehension of *who* vs. *which NP* dependencies in Croatian aphasics can be made in several ways. For instance:

(a) The Chain Disruption Hypothesis. A proposal according to which binding chains involved in *which NP* dependencies are disrupted, while government chains, involved in *who* type of *wh*-dependencies, are preserved in Broca's aphasics (Hickok & Avrutin, 1996), does not account for the Croatian data, where either both types of chains are comprehended, or they are not comprehended at all. Thus, this proposal does not explain the lack of difference in comprehension of *who* vs. *which NP* dependencies in Croatian Broca's aphasics.

(b) The TBA account (R-strategy). A proposal based on R-strategy, which requires that a theta role be assigned to a referential NP without a theta-role "by its linear position" (Grodzinsky, 1995, p. 221), does

not explain the Croatian data. Since there is no difference in comprehension of referential (*which* NP) vs. non-referential (*who*) NPs in Croatian, the R-strategy, if applied, is used for both, referential and non-referential *wh*-phrases, or it is not used at all by Croatian aphasics. Thus, this account cannot explain the lack of difference in comprehension of *who* vs. *which NP* questions found in Croatian Broca's aphasics.

(c) Semantic Representation-Based Account. A proposal based on differences in semantic representations of *who* and *which NP* dependencies suggests that *which NP* dependencies are semantically more difficult because they involve an additional predication relation to compute (Tait et al., 1995, Thompson et al., 1999). However, since no differences were found in *who* vs. *which NP* dependencies in the Croatian Broca's data, we can conclude that an additional semantic predication involved in *which NP* questions does not affect comprehension of *who* vs. *which NP* to such an extent that it causes significant differences in their comprehension. Therefore, this proposal is not supported by the Croatian data.

(d) Integration of Syntax and Discourse. This proposal is built on the idea of processing differences between *who* and *which NP* dependencies (Hickok & Avrutin, 1993). It suggests that *which NP* dependencies are more difficult to process than *who* dependencies because they require not only syntactic processing, but also discourse processing, and that it is precisely the integration of syntax and discourse that imposes additional processing load (Avrutin, 2000). Since Broca's aphasic patients have depleted processing resources, as shown for instance by Zurif et al. (1993), they have difficulty processing structures that impose such excessive processing load. This view, however, runs against the idea that *which NP* questions are actually easier to comprehend, because they are D-linked and thus there is only a limited set of potential referents from which to choose. This proposal, like other proposals mentioned above, does not explain the data from Croatian Broca's aphasics.

8.3.2 Subject vs. Object

Several elements can be discerned and analyzed in the search for a structural explanation for the lack of subject-object asymmetry in the Croatian data.

(a) Canonicity. Although Croatian has a relatively free word order, it is possible to discern a typical word order: S + AUX + V + O. Given that the subject comes first, an explanation based on canonicity would predict better comprehension of dependencies with extraction from subject position. Since the Croatian data show lack of asymmetry, an explanation from canonicity does not apply.

(b) Distance. Given that the distance between subjects and their traces is smaller than the distance between objects and their traces in *wh*-dependencies (since the subject position is closer to the sentence-initial *wh*-word), we would expect better comprehension of structures with subject extraction than structures with extractions from object position. However, the lack of asymmetry found in Croatian Broca's aphasics suggests that the syntactic concept of distance between antecedents and their traces cannot explain the Croatian data.

Thus, previous analyses of comprehension of subject and object *wh*-dependencies in English, whether structural or processing-based, cannot explain the Croatian data.

8.4 Morphological Explanation of the Lack of Asymmetry in Broca's Aphasics

Given the structural differences between English and Croatian, and the findings on Serbo-Croatian Broca's aphasics' sensitivity to inflectional morphology (Smith & Mimica, 1984; Lukatela et al., 1988), it is reasonable to resort to morphology in search for an explanation of the lack of asymmetry in the Croatian data. From the morphological point of view, *tko* and *koji NP* are equally informative with respect to their indicating the grammatical function of the moved *wh*-word in a sentence. Subject and object forms of both *tko* and *koji NP* have case endings that unambiguously indicate their grammatical functions[1]. Assuming that the parser has full access to grammatical information, it is actually not surprising that there are no differences in aphasics' comprehension of *who* vs. *which NP* dependencies in Croatian. Thus, the pattern predicted from

[1] An exception here are *which NPs* containing nouns in neuter, where there is ambiguity in Nominative vs. Accusative case marking: *Koje lane je pratilo zebru?* "Which fawn followed the zebra?" vs. *Koje lane je zebra pratila?* "Which fawn did the zebra follow?" Here the case-cuing strategy would consist in relying on the case marking on the second noun for preliminary theta-role assignment.

morphology would be *subject equals object*, i.e., *no asymmetry*, which explains the Croatian Broca's aphasics' data.

If *who* dependencies, being non-D-linked, are harder to process than D-linked *which NP* dependencies (it is easier to pick an entity from a limited than from an unlimited set of entities), then perhaps the asymmetry between *tko* and *koji NP* is balanced out by the case endings which unambiguously signal grammatical role of a *wh*-word, enabling the parser to temporarily assign thematic roles. Alternatively, we could assume that *who* dependencies are easier to process, because they do not obey discourse requirements in addition to the requirements of syntax (e.g., they do not have to be "integrated" in discourse in the same ways as *which NP* structures) (Avrutin, 2000), and since there is one more predication relation involved in *which NP* dependencies (Tait et al., 1995). In that case, one could argue that the additional morphological features contained in the inflectional ending in *koji NP* in Croatian (gender and number) balance out processing, resulting in equal or close to equal comprehension of *wh*-dependencies in Croatian aphasics. Thus, if there are syntactic differences between *tko* and *koji* NP, as discussed in section 8.3.1, the morphological features conveyed by the inflectional endings of fronted *wh*-words have the potential to compensate for them, predicting the equal or close to equal *tko/koji* comprehension. Croatian Broca's aphasics, as has already been noticed (Smith & Mimica, 1984; Lukatela et al., 1988), have preserved ability to use that information.

8.5 The Research Questions Revisited

This study investigated the question of whether Croatian speaking Broca's aphasics exhibit the subject-object asymmetry in comprehension of *who* and *which NP* dependencies that was found in English speaking Broca's patients. Three possible outcomes with regard to the experimental results were identified:

A. There is no asymmetry in comprehension of subject vs. object *who/which* dependencies in Croatian Broca's aphasics.
B. There is asymmetry in comprehension of subject vs. object *who/which* dependencies in Croatian aphasics, and it matches the asymmetric pattern found in English speaking Broca's aphasics.
C. There is asymmetry, but it does not match the asymmetric pattern reported for the English speaking Broca's aphasics.

The experimental results have shown a lack of asymmetry in Croatian Broca's aphasics, thereby confirming prediction A. Predictions B and C were not confirmed for the Croatian Broca's aphasics, but some asymmetry was found in the cases with mixed nonfluent aphasia. Mixed nonfluent aphasia resembles Broca's aphasia, but it has a more pronounced comprehension deficit. Thus, the Croatian data represent an excellent opportunity to learn more about the patterns of comprehension of *wh*-dependencies in these patients.

8.6 Patterns of Comprehension in Cases with Nonfluent Mixed Aphasia

8.6.1 Objects-Better: Direct Questions, Embedded Questions, Long-Distance Questions, and Relative Clauses

Aphasic participants T.P., B.R., and J.Z. differ from the three Broca's aphasics in their ability to comprehend the tested *wh*-dependencies. While there were no statistically significant differences in Broca's aphasics' comprehension of subject vs. object *wh*-dependencies, what is remarkable about the results of patients with mixed nonfluent aphasia is a pattern of significantly better comprehension of *wh-s*tructures extracted from object position compared to those extracted from subject position, as shown in Table 7-10. Explanations based on filler-gap distance or canonicity cannot explain this comprehension pattern, as shown in Section 8.3.2. However, the pattern can be explained in terms of compensatory strategies, as it seems to reflect reliance on case cueing.

Gleason, Goodglass, Green, Ackerman and Hyde (1975) argued that not only direct evidence of deficit in aphasia is relevant, such as omissions, substitutions, simplifications of structures and so on; adaptive or compensatory strategies are also informative and relevant. Even though they may differ from patient to patient, such strategies are more often found in patients with more severe aphasia. As an example of such strategy at work, Gleason et al. reported that 42 initial vocatives were produced by four severe aphasics, while only 13 initial vocatives were produced by four mild aphasics. The Croatian data also show that patients with a more pronounced comprehension deficit, such as B.R. and J.Z., relied more on a compensatory strategy based on case cueing.

One model of grammatical processing that explains sentence comprehension based on cueing is the competition model (Bates & MacWhinney, 1987; MacWhinney, 1987).

8.6.1.1 The Competition Model

The competition model was developed to explain cross-linguistic differences in processing primarily in child language, but it has also been used to study language processing in normal and brain-damaged adults (Bates et al., 2001). The model is based on the idea that processing in structurally different languages reflects the structural differences among languages and that different languages rely on different types of information as cues in sentence processing.

The model assumes that the language processor will choose which information to attend to in determining sentence meaning based on a cue's strength. The strength of a cue is determined by its availability, reliability, and its processing cost. A cue is high in availiability if it is available for assessing "the underlying function", and high in reliability if it is not misleading or ambiguous in signaling the correct interpretation (Kempe & MacWhinney, 1999, p. 130). Cue validity depends on cue cost in interpretation: if processing even a highly informative cue is very costly, then such a cue may be abandoned and replaced by a cue with less information value. The cue cost depends on perceivability and assignability of the cue. Perceivability refers to the ease with which a cue is detectable, while assignability denotes the ease with which a cue can be assigned in sentence processing (Bates & MacWhinney, 1987). An example of a cue with high assignability is case marking in Turkish: as soon as the suffix that marks a case on a noun is classified, a thematic role of that noun is assigned.

While English typically relies on the word order cue, Italian on the verb agreement cue, Hungarian, like Turkish, relies on the case marking cues. Crucially, the competition model assumes parallel processing of various information types, and so in addition to the strongest cue, each language relies on other cues. As an example, languages such as Spanish, Italian and German rely on the animacy cue much more than English or Hungarian. Under certain circumstances and when more dominant cues that are typically available in Spanish, Italian and German are absent, the language processor may rely on the animacy cue in sentence processing (Kempe & MacWhinney, 1999).

Consider the preposition *a* in Spanish. It has weak cue validity, and yet evidence indicates that it can guide sentence comprehension. More specifically, the preposition *a* can have several different meanings and thus its reliability is low. It also has low availability, because it is used only with animate direct objects. However, despite its weak cue validity, the preposition *a* has "an extremely high contrast validity… Among normal speakers, in fact, it is the most overriding cue in determining semantic role" (Benedet et al., 1998, p. 332).

The competition model predicts that the strongest cues appear earlier than weaker cues in child language and that such cues are better retained in impaired language. In contrast, the weaker cues are first to break down under stress. For example, in English word order is a strong cue while morphology is a weak cue, whereas the distribution of cue strength is opposite in Italian, German, or Croatian where morphology is strong and word order is a relatively poor cue. Sensitivity of 2 year old Serbian/Croatian-speaking children to case marking is another example of a strong cue at work (Bates & MacWhinney, 1987).

In addition to the relevance of individual cues in sentence processing, research on healthy elderly persons has shown that assignment of Agent-Patient roles in a sentence typically depends on a convergence of cues. The reliance on cue convergence is even more pronounced in aphasic population (Smith & Mimica, 1984), where cue validity may be affected because the processing system is under stress or limited in storage capacity (Bates & MacWhinney, 1987; Benedet et al., 1998; Bates et al, 2001). In a study on comprehension of simple declarative sentences with Agent-Patient relations in Serbo-Croatian speaking Broca's aphasics, Smith and Mimica (1984) have shown that convergence of two or more cues, which all indicated the Agent role of a specific noun, led to comprehension that "resembled that of normal control subjects" (p. 286). In contrast, when there was only a single cue, even if it was the strong cue such as case marking, these speakers' comprehension was less consistent.

The competition model explains the pattern of better comprehension of object than subject *wh*-dependencies in Croatian patients with mixed nonfluent aphasia. Based on previous research on case morphology and thematic roles in Serbian (Katz, Rexer & Peter, 1995), Kljajevic and Murasugi (2010) proposed that Nominative and Accusative in Croatian have different cue validity. Namely, Nominative case and Accusative case differ in reliability, with the latter being more reliable than the former. Since Nominative can be ambiguous with regard to the thematic role that is assigned to the noun it marks, it is less reliable than Accusative, which is typically associated with the direct object and with the role of Patient.

However, some researchers claim that in Serbian, and also in Croatian, Accusative actually has more thematic roles than Nominative, which would mean that it is thematically more ambiguous than Nominative, and so more difficult to process. However, since "the accusative is the case that encodes the direct object of a verb" and "the direct object encodes the patient by definition" (Blake, 1994, p. 134), the thematic richness of

Accusative is perhaps more relevant in other, less typical contexts, unlike those tested in the present study. The following represents a hierarchy of accessibility to subject, and also to object (with the exception of the agent, which cannot be expressed by object) (Blake, 1994, p. 92):

(15) Agent > Patient > Recipient > Beneficiary > Instrument > Location > Temporal

Furthermore, Accusative has a more perceivable marking, which allows that a thematic role of Patient be assigned as soon as the marking is identified. Note however that the Nominative form *koji* is also ambiguous with regard to gender: *koji pas* (singular) vs. *koji psi* (plural), which is not the case with its form in Accusative: *kojeg psa* (singular) vs. *koje pse* (plural).

Thus, a convergence of cues fused in the suffix that also indicates Accusative makes it more perceivable and therefore easier to processes than Nominative.

8.6.1.2 Evidence from Spanish

A recent study with elderly native speakers of Spanish (Kljajevic & Fratini, 2011) compared comprehension of *wh*-dependencies in healthy elderly (n = 11), elderly with a mild cognitive impairment (MCI) (n = 10) and healthy young participants as a control group (n = 18) (Section 7.10). While healthy elderly and young participants performed above chance on all 4 types of direct questions (subject *who,* object *who,* subject *which NP,* and object *which NP*), the group of elderly with MCI showed a different comprehension pattern. They comprehended above chance direct object *who* questions, while their comprehension of direct subject *who* questions was at chance. Accuracy of understanding the four types of sentences was analyzed in a mixed-model, repeated-measures analysis of variance (ANOVA) with a between-subject factor comparing groups (MCI, healthy elderly, young) and within-subjects factors comparing the extraction site in a sentence (subject, object) and the type of *wh*-word (*who, which*). This test design was combined with Tukey's test as a post-hoc test. There were statistically significant differences in the participants' overall sentence comprehension between the groups (F (2,36) = 37.844, $p < .001 < .05$), and further analyses by Tukey's test showed that there were significant differences in the comprehension between the young and MCI group (p = .0005), and between the normal healthy elderly and MCI group (p = .0005). In both cases the MCI group had lower accuracy. The difference between the young and healthy elderly was not significant. The main effect of extraction site (subject/object) was significant (F (1,36) = 4.479. $p < .05$), reflecting better comprehension of object structures.

Like in Croatian, the distance between the moved *wh*-word and its trace differs in Spanish subject and object direct questions, as shown in (16) and (17):

(16) ¿Quién$_i$ t_i comió una naranja?
"Who ate an orange?"

(17) ¿A quién$_i$ mordió$_j$ el perrito t_j t_i ?
"Who did the puppy bit?"

Given that the distance between the moved *wh*-word and its trace is longer in object questions, as in (17), than in subject questions, as in (16), we would expect processing of object structures to be more demanding. Thus, the finding from Spanish that object-extracted direct *who* questions were better comprehended than subject-extracted direct *who* questions is not in line with the accounts that explain processing in terms of filler-gap distance.

However, the finding can be explained in terms of a strategy based on syntactic cueing: direct object questions are introduced by a PP in Spanish (e.g., *a quién, a qué*), beginning with the preposition *a*, as in (17). The preposition *a* in Spanish marks animate direct objects, serving as a cue to predict and assign a preliminary thematic role of Patient to the initial constituent in object-extracted sentences, such as (17). The data from Spanish show that this information was utilized by the MCI group in the comprehension of direct object *who* questions.

On the other hand, the MCI group comprehended below chance the object-extracted direct *which NP* questions, such as (18).

(18) ¿A qué niño besó la abuela?
"Which boy did the grandma kiss?"

This finding supports the claim that *which NP* questions may be more difficult to process than *who* questions, perhaps because they require integration of syntax and discourse (Avrutin, 2000). Thus, even though the preposition *a* was available to guide the comprehension of direct object *which NP* questions through cueing, the overall processing demands were higher than the available resources, and comprehension failed. Spanish *qué,* unlike Croatian *koji,* lacks additional morphological features that would facilitate processing.

Thus, the evidence from Spanish indicates that the *objects-better* pattern of comprehension of *wh*-dependencies is available in other languages and populations, at least in structures introduced by non-D-linked *wh*-words.

8.6.2 Subjects-Better: Passivized Questions and Extended Embedded Questions

While Croatian patients with mixed nonfluent aphasia B.R. and J.Z. showed a relatively robust pattern of better comprehension of object- than subject-extracted direct, embedded, and long-distance *wh*-questions and relative clauses, they exhibited the opposite pattern in their comprehension of passivized and extended embedded *who/which NP* questions. Computational demands of these structures in Croatian are presented in Sections 8.2.1 and 8.2.2, where it was suggested that the processing demands of these two types of structures may differ from the processing demands associated with other tested structures. B.R.'s (Section 7.6.3) and J.Z.'s (Section 7.7.3) comprehension patterns revealed their better comprehension of subject than object extractions from these structures, which indicates that the case cueing strategy used in other conditions was not suitable for passivized and extended embedded questions.

Languages typically use passive as a marked choice for subject: in passive constructions the direct object has been advanced to subject, whereas the subject has been demoted to a "peripheral relation" (Blake, 1994, p. 89). Thus, there is a mismatch between grammatical functions and thematic roles, as shown in passive questions given in Table 6-4.4. For instance, in the subject *who* question *Tko je ritnut od zebre?* the *wh*-pronoun *tko* is in Nominative, but it carries the role of Patient, while *od zebre* is Genitive and it carries the thematic role of Agent. The role of Patient is associated with the less marked Nominative case, while Genitive is associated with the role of Agent. The genitive case, however, is not a typical Agent, and so the case cueing strategy would fail to assign the correct thematic role in this case.

Passivized object questions begin with the Genitive *wh*-phrase, which signals the role of Agent, while the role of Patient is encoded in Nominative. Since these are not typical *case-grammatical function-thematic role* associations, they require processing strategies different from case cueing. One such strategy may be reliance on the most typical word order. Croatian, as shown in Chapter 3, is a subject-first language and so the strategy of picking a subject over object interpretation could have led to the *subjects-better* pattern. As shown in Section 8.6.1.1, when the strongest cue in a language is not available, as for instance when the direct object and the role of Patient are not indicated by Accusative, the processor relies on other cues that are available (word order, verb agreement, etc.).

Similarly, B.R. and J.Z. could have relied on these other cues, mainly on word order, in their comprehension of extended embedded questions, where due to excessive WM demands imposed by the additional phrase(s) in these structures the case cueing strategy may have been ineffective. In conclusion, both case cueing and reliance on word order contribute to comprehension by reducing the SWM load: they allow the parser to immediately begin minimal phrase building and interpretation, without having to wait to encounter the gap. When these strategies are not applied, less favourable comprehension results.

CHAPTER NINE

CONCLUSION

9.1 Summary of Findings

This study investigated comprehension of *wh*-dependencies in 8 Croatian aphasics. Three of them were Broca's aphasics, and four patients had mixed aphasia. One patient had residual anomic aphasia, after recovering from transcortical-sensory aphasia.

The main goal of the study was to determine whether Croatian aphasics, especially those diagnosed with Broca's aphasia, have difficulty comprehending *wh*-dependencies, i.e., structures formed with *who* and *which NP*. Four experiments were designed, containing syntactic structures of graded degrees of complexity: direct, embedded, long-distance and passivized questions as well as relative clauses. Two types of long-distance questions were tested: those with the preposition *za* and those without *za*. Three types of embedded questions were tested: non-extended embedded questions, embedded questions with 1 extension (PP) and embedded questions with 2 extensions. Each type of syntactic structure was tested for subjects and objects, for both *who* and *which NP* (see Table 6-3). The same material was administered to three control subjects. In addition to the experiments, the patients were administered evaluative tests: the Digit Span Backwards, RCPM, the BDAE and Supplementary Language subtests pertaining to auditory comprehension. The results of two sets of measures are in accord.

The main finding of the study is that, unlike English-speaking Broca's aphasics, Croatian speaking Broca's aphasics do not exhibit the pattern of asymmetric comprehension of *wh*-dependencies. This was also found in the patient diagnosed with anomia (S.T.), in one patient with mixed nonfluent aphasia (T.P.), and in the patient with mixed fluent aphasia (K.S.), who, unlike the others with this pattern, showed chance comprehension on most conditions. The *no asymmetry* pattern was then explained by means of a structural and processing approach: Croatian uses information conveyed by inflectional endings of a moved *wh*-phrase (case marking), which facilitates comprehension processes by enabling establishment of grammatical functions and temporary assignment of thematic roles. Since these morphological tools are not available in English, processing of *wh*-dependencies differs in two languages.

However, some asymmetry was found in patients with mixed nonfluent aphasia B.R. and J.Z. Their comprehension pattern consists in better comprehension of object than subject extractions in direct, embedded, long-distance questions and relative clauses, and better comprehension of subject compared to object extractions in extended embedded and passivized questions. The *objects better* pattern was explained in terms of a comprehension strategy based on case cueing and competition model.

Another finding of the study pertains to the lesion-deficit relationship. Although we cannot deduce from the Croatian data which specific brain area(s) needs to be damaged for a deficit in comprehension of *wh*-dependencies to appear (all the patients had large and sometimes multiple lesions), the evidence suggests that the same pattern of comprehension of *wh*-dependencies (no asymmetry, objects-better) was associated with different distributions of lesions (cortical, cortical-subcortical, subcortical). The role of subcortical structures in language function remains unclear (Ojemann, 1991) and even less is known about individual variability in functional neuroplastic post-stroke changes. Crucially, their lesions still allowed the patients to use a comprehension strategy to differing extents. This indicates the importance of clinical data to the study of mechanisms of syntactic processing.

There are few theoretical implications of this study, pertaining to processing of complex syntax. The patterns of spared vs. impaired comprehension more generally indicate that the language processing system is modular and that its components may dissociate after brain damage.

9.2 Theoretical Implications

One of the research questions of this study pertains to the underlying cognitive mechanisms implicated in the processing of *wh*-dependencies (see Section 6.2). More specifically, based on the results of experiments and subject profiles in 8 aphasic patients, the study tries to deduce the impact of these components on comprehension in Broca's aphasics. In a wider sense, it extends the context of the study of *wh*-dependencies from a specific syntactic problem within the language architecture to the functional architecture of cognition, thereby touching upon the localization and modularity hypotheses.

Linguistic theories that have tried to explain syntactic processing within the modularity framework mostly adopt the idea of informational encapsulation of modules, i.e., modules are informationally specific and closed systems, which do not allow penetration of information from other modules. Informational encapsulation is problematic, because it does not allow free flow and exchange of information among different cognitive modules. The concept of interface modules that is emerging from the recent, more flexible proposals[1] on cognitive architecture (Jackendoff, 2000, 2002) seems to answer the question of how different cognitive domains, that are engaged in processing of a "single" task such as sentence comprehension, communicate information among themselves, resulting in successful performance of that task (Van der Zee & Nikanne, 2000; Jackendoff, 1997, 2000, 2002; Platzack, 2000; Slack, 2000).

9.2.1 Modularity: Classical vs. Representational Approach

The idea that the language faculty is a component of the human mind/brain (Chomsky, 1975, 1981) fits into the context of the modularity hypothesis, as defined and debated by cognitive scientists and linguists[2]: the cognitive architecture is modular, i.e., it consists of functionally independent systems (modules), such as language or vision (Fodor, 1983), and the central processes. A cognitive system is a module in this classical sense if it is informationally encapsulated, domain specific, innately specified, hardwired (neurally specific), fast, mandatory, autonomous, and not assembled. The listed characteristics, however, are possible features of a module, and, in order to be defined as a module, a component of the mind does not have to have all of them (Coltheart, 2001).

Nevertheless, the most important aspect of a module in the classical approach is its informational encapsulation—a characteristic that prevents a module's activities and outputs from being influenced by information that belongs to another module or non-modular part of cognition (i.e., central processes). For instance, according to this view, the syntactic processing of language is encapsulated from nonsyntactic information:

---

[1] The concept of cognitive interfaces is becoming increasingly important to both classical symbolic and modular as well as non-symbolic and non-modular theories of cognition (van der Zee & Nikanne, 2000).

[2] The term *modularity* in neuroscience refers to the *brain's* structure and its systems.

> … I know of no convincing evidence that syntactic parsing is ever guided by the subject's appreciation of pragmatic context or of 'real world' background (Fodor, 1983, p. 78).

It has been debated whether on-line (real-time) syntactic processing can be isolated from other types of information present in language processing, such as semantic, prosodic, or pragmatic information, for the purposes of analysis. However, as Jackendoff has pointed out, rigid informational encapsulation of a system renders its content (information) "useless to the rest of the brain" (Jackendoff, 2000, p. 19), which in the case of a syntactic module means that it is impossible to connect syntax with semantics, as in assigning preliminary thematic roles in the course of building a minimal clausal structure. Thus, unlike modular accounts of sentence comprehension, which assume that the information internal to the semantic module is not available to or employed by the syntactic module, the representatives of the interactive approach argue for the simultaneous and interactive use of syntactic and semantic information in the process of building sentence representation. Moreover, semantic information may trigger a specific syntactic analysis (Stowe, 1989).

Many researchers understand language modularity in terms of innateness, localization and domain specificity (Bates, 2001). The innateness hypothesis postulates that the human language capacity is innate. The localization hypothesis, which postulates that language is processed by a few language-specialized brain areas, has been revised due to new findings provided by neuroimaging techniques, such as PET, fMRI, and MEG. The new findings are not consistent with the classical approach, according to which there exist language areas or language zones (Zurif et al., 1993; Zurif, 1995). They rather suggest that language is widely distributed in the brain (Kutas et al., 2000), which is enabled by multiple relative specializations of different brain areas (Keller et al., 2001). Broca's area is one example of such functional overlap or multiple relative specializations. Thus, the localization question has not been solved; it has just acquired a new dimension, weakening the classical modularity hypothesis and providing space in which to search for potential arguments supporting more interactivity within cognition.

Furthermore, it is not clear how to explain functional reorganization of language in a post-stroke brain within the strict localizationist hypothesis. Namely, after a specific function has been compromised due to brain damage, brain areas that are not typically involved in that function may be recruited to support tasks associated with that function. The question of how the reorganization of language happens in post-stroke brain has been extensively debated in the literature. Recent evidence indicates that there exist specific temporal and spatial dynamics of language reorganization (Saur, Lange, Baumgaertner, Schraknepper, Willmes, et al., 2006). According to Saur et al. (2006), three distinct temporal post-stroke phases—acute, subacute and chronic—are associated with different spatial patterns of brain activation. More specifically, their longitudinal fMRI study with post-stroke aphasic patients showed that there was little perilesional activation in the acute phase, the subacute phase was associated mostly with activation of the right hemisphere homologous areas, while in the chronic phase the function reshifted to the left hemisphere in the aphasics who exhibited language improvement. It is not clear how these changes affect the rules of grammar and the mechanisms involved in their processing. Thus, although language function is in principle localizable, these findings cannot be captured by the strict localizationist hypothesis.

Another pertinent concept of modularity is domain specificity, which is based on the assumption that modules are informationally exclusive. The assumption seems too strong, given that domain is a multilevel concept: a system can be specific at one level and yet very general at another (Bates, 2001). For instance, language tasks, knowledge of language and its representations are unique to the domain of language. However, it is less clear whether the mechanisms involved in their processing and the neural substrate supporting them are also language specific. A growing body of evidence indicates that it is not likely that some neural tissue serves exclusively for language processing, which furthermore requires resources from other domains (memory, attention, etc.). Consequently, it requires processing mechanisms that are capable of using these different resources simultaneously, processing different types of information and dealing with the constraints on information linking at the same time.

A similar insight has been used as a basis for the representational version of modularity proposed by Jackendoff (1997, 2000, 2002). Jackendoff postulates two types of modules: integrative modules, which integrate information within particular levels of representation, and interface modules, which communicate information among the integrative modules (Jackendoff, 2000). Thus, instead of a faculty-size language module, the representational modularity hypothesis postulates chains of integrative and interface modules, allowing "a single level of representation to be fed simultaneously by multiple interface processors" (Jackendoff, 2000, p. 17). Crucially, such modules differ with regard to the extent to which they are informationally encapsulated and domain specific.

The concept of cognitive interface is the key notion underlying representational modularity: cognitive interfaces, in contrast to the classical modules, are not restricted to one domain. Instead, they are connected to two integrative domains, enabling performance of tasks that require simultaneous involvement of two domains. Thus, in Jackendoff's view, although interface modules are still domain specific, their domain specificity is extended by the interface requirements for connecting with two independent cognitive systems involved in the processing of particular information.

Unlike the classical approach, representational modularity allows an incomplete representation to activate another module that can use that information. For instance, in a model of language comprising phonology, syntax and propositional structure as integrative modules, the phonology-syntax interface module and the syntax-propositional interface may pass information between the integrative modules without having to wait for the representations to be complete (Jackendoff, 2000). This intermodular feedback is important for the theories of processing that try to explain effects of nonsyntactic information on parsing and rely on the assumption of incremental sentence processing.

9.2.2 SWM: An Interface Module?

Both intra- and inter-modular connectedness is required in language processing. The former is captured by the models of grammar in which there is a level of phonological, syntactic, semantic/conceptual, and discourse representation. For instance, syntactic theories such as GB assume a modular grammar. The latter can be exemplified by the role of the memory subsystem employed in syntactic computations that has been termed *syntactic working memory* (Lewis, 1999; Fiebach et al., 2001, 2002). The idea is that SWM is an interface module enabling temporary storage and manipulation of intermediate syntactic representations that emerge in the course of building full sentential representations. Given the evidence on the involvement of SWM in the processing of musical syntax and other hierarchical representations, one could speculate that the concept of SWM is not necessarily language-specific and that it can actually function as a cognitive interface module for other domains as well. This idea is supported by the neuroimaging evidence indicating involvement of Broca's area in a variety of tasks, including action, music and so on (Section 2.3.3) and it is theoretically compatible with representational modularity:

> Suppose there are brain areas for whose use more than one integrative module competes, and which shift allegiances depending on attention. Such an area would be in a position to detect and record fortuitous

> coincidences in pattern between two modules that are capable of using it. It might therefore be possible for it to *develop* into an interface processor without having any special use for that purpose wired into it from the start (Jackendoff, 2000, p. 22).

However, how exactly SWM contributes to processing in a wider sense and whether it involves syntax of language only are topics for future research.

9.3 Future Research

At this point, the distinction between the questions of whether Broca's area is indeed the locus of certain types of syntactic operations, such as those related to syntactic displacement, or a specific aspect of WM employed for the purposes of these syntactic operations, starts losing its sharp edges. The focus is shifting from the question of whether Broca's area subserves syntax in general, only syntactic processing involved in syntactic movement, or SWM instead, to the questions of what other parts of the brain are implicated in syntactic processing and issues on how language processors interface with WM and attention. Nevertheless, the search will continue to find a functional definition of Broca's area, for which evidence from aphasia remains indispensable (Chatterjee, 2005).

In contrast, the distinction between *where* exactly in the brain and *when* in the course of processing the breakdown in syntactic comprehension in Broca's patients occurs is sharper then ever. Computation of dependency relations in syntax requires language external resources, such as WM, to handle manipulations on intermediate representations in time. Broca's aphasics experience breakdown in these processes somewhere before the final result is reached. Observing *when* exactly the processing crashes provides an excellent opportunity to study how comprehension processes unfold in time. This is becoming increasingly important, as evidence from structurally different languages indicates that different information may be used by the parser to guide processing in different languages (e.g., word order, case markings, verb agreement, and so on).

Choosing between the two perspectives – *where in the brain* vs. *when* processing crashes - has theoretical and methodological consequences for neurocognitive study of syntactic processing. Theoretically, the former intends to solve the localization question for syntax (*Where in the brain do syntactic processes occur?*), while the latter focuses on timing (*How do these processes unfold in time*?). Given the different perspectives and complexity of both questions, research on comprehension deficits needs to employ to a greater extent on-line investigation of the processes involved, employing techniques such as fMRI, ERP, and MEG. The fMRI method is necessary because of its high spatial resolution, while the high temporal resolution of the latter two methods enables observation of temporal processing patterns. The impact of neuroimaging on our understanding of the neural correlates of language, functionality of Broca's area and its multiple relative specializations has been debated in the literature (e.g., Fedorenko and Kanwisher, 2009; Grodzinsky, 2010; Pulvermüller, 2010). However, due to the findings mainly from neuroimaging the search for anatomical loci of highly specialized language areas has shifted towards the question of how to capture the spatial and temporal dynamics of language as a distributed function (Kljajevic, 2011a). As a result, more dynamic neurocognitive models of language have been proposed (e.g., Friederici, 1998; Hickok & Poeppel, 2000, 2004, 2007). Finally, stimulation methods such as Transcranial Magnetic Stimulation (TMS) and transcranial Direct Current Stimulation (tDCS), in addition to serving as an excellent choice for studying virtual lesions, have shown a great potential in rehabilitation of language (Naeser, Martin, Nicholas, Baker, Seekins, et al., 2005), providing new insights on how the brain reorganizes language after a stroke.

As discussed in the book, research on aphasia thus far has mostly been based on behavioral off-line and sometimes on-line methods. Sentence-picture matching, act-out tasks, and grammaticality-judgment tasks are all off-line behavioral methods in the sense that they are not concerned with subjects' real-time responses as they perform a certain task. While off-line paradigms are acceptable for testing general comprehension of sentences (Ueno, 2003), research on the processing of traces of dislocated syntactic elements needs application of on-line methods (Zurif et al., 1993). Furthermore, behavioral methods are not informative enough with regards to which neural structures these processes are based on (Müller et al., 1997). For example, although behavioral cross-modal priming experiments show that an antecedent is reactivated as soon as the parser reaches its trace, they cannot show "how the structural configurations internal to the sentence elicit WM costs" (Fiebach et al., 2002, p. 251). The methods based on reaction-time measurement cannot be reliably used with aphasic patients when investigating their sentence processing on-line, because these patients often cannot make fast and accurate movements (e.g., pressing a button) and it is precisely these movements that are being measured as indicators of on-line processing (Müller et al., 1997).

Techniques that overcome these limitations by enabling measurement of the brain's activity throughout the processing are ERP and MEG. Although ERP and MEG studies of aphasic language processing are still rare, these methods have the potential to untangle many problems that exist at the moment, in particular if combined with fMRI. One can hope that these methods will become increasingly available in hospitals and accessible to researchers, because insights on how damaged brain processes and recovers language are necessarily limited if based on a single method (Ojemann, 1991). Since methodology often shapes theory, with the methodological limits stretching upon the theory itself, an ideal approach would combine behavioral with neural on-line methods (ERP, MEG, fMRI). Research on comprehension deficits in Broca's aphasic patients, including the topic addressed in this book, would certainly benefit from such combination of methods.

BIBLIOGRAPHY

Alexander, M.P., Naeser, M.A., Palumbo, C. (1990). Broca's area aphasias: aphasias after lesions including the frontal operculum. *Neurology, 40,* 353-362.

Amunts, K., Schleicher, A., Bürgel, U., Mohlberg, H., Uylings, H.B.M. & Zilles, K. (1999). Broca's Region Revisited: Cytoarchitecture and Intersubject Variability. The *Journal of Comparative Neurology, 412*, 319-341.

Amunts, K., Schleicher, A., Ditterich, A. & Zilles, K. (2003). Broca's region: Cytoarchitectonic Asymmetry and Developmental Changes. *The Journal of Comparative Neurology, 465*, 72-89.

Amunts, K., Schleicher, A. & Zilles, K. (2004). Outstanding language competence and cytoarchitecture in Broca's speech region. *Brain and Language, 89*, 346-353.

Amunts, K. & Zilles, K. (2006). A Multimodal Analysis of Structure and Function of Broca's Area. In: Grodzinsky, Y. & Amunts, K. (Eds.), *Broca's Region* (17-30). Oxford: Oxford University Press.

Ardila, A. (2010). A proposed reinterpretation and reclassification of aphasic syndromes. *Aphasiology, 24(3),* 363-394.

Avrutin, S. (1999). *Development of the Syntax-Discourse Interface*. Dordrecht: Kluwer Academic Publishers.

—. (2000). Comprehension of Discourse-Linked and Non-Discourse-Linked Questions by Children and Broca's Aphasics. In: Grodzinsky, Y., Saphiro, L. & Swinney, D. (Eds.), *Language and the Brain* (pp. 295-313). San Diego: Academic Press.

Baddeley, A. (1990). *Human Memory. Theory and Practice*. Boston: Allyn and Bacon.

—. (2000). Working Memory: The Interface between Memory and Cognition. In: Gazzaniga, M.S. (Ed.), *Cognitive Neuroscience. A Reader.* Oxford: Blackwell Publishers.

—. (2003). Working Memory: Looking Back and Looking Forward. *Nature Reviews Neuroscience, 4(10),* 829-839.

Badecker, W. & Caramazza, A. (1985). On considerations of method and theory governing the use of clinical categories in neurolinguistics and cognitive neuropsychology: the case against agrammatism. *Cognition, 20*, 97-125.

Baldo, J. & Dronkers, N. (2006). The role of inferior parietal and inferior frontal cortex in working memory. *Neuropsychology, 20,* 529-538.

Balogh, J. & Grodzinsky, Y. (1996). Varieties of passives in agrammatic Broca's aphasia: theta grids, arguments, and referentiality. In: Whitacker, H. (Ed.), Academy of Aphasia. London: Academic Press.

Balogh, J.E. & Grodzinsky, Y. (2000). Levels of Linguistic Representation in Broca's Aphasia: Implicitness and Referentiality of Arguments. In: Bastianse,

R. & Grodzinsky, Y. (Eds.), *Grammatical Disorders in Aphasia: A Neurolinguistic Perspective.* London: Whur Publishers.

Baretta, A. & Munn, A. (1998). Double-Agents and Trace-Deletion in Agrammatism. *Brain and Language, 65*, 404-421.

Basso, A. (2003). *Aphasia and its Therapy*. Oxford: Oxford University Press.

Bastiaanse R. Broca's Aphasia: (1995). A Syntactic and/or a Morphological Disorder? A Case Study. *Brain and Language, 48,* 1-32

Bates, E. (2001). Modularity, Domain Specificity and the Development of Language. In: Edited by Bechtel, W., Mandik, P., Mundale, J. &. Stufflebeam, R.S. *Philosophy and the Neurosciences. A Reader* (pp. 134-152). Oxford: Blackwell Publishers.

Bates, E., & MacWhinney, B. (1987). Competition, variation, and language learning. In B. MacWhinney (Ed.), *Mechanisms of Language Acquisition* (pp. 157–193). Hillsdale, NJ: Lawrence Erlbaum Associates, Publishers.

Benedet, M., Christiansen, J. & Goodglass, H. (1998). A cross-linguistic study of grammatical morphology in Spanish and English speaking agrammatic patients. *Cortex, 34*, 309–336.

Ben-Shachar M., Palti D. & Grodzinsky Y. (2004). Neural Correlates of Syntactic Movement: Converging Evidence from Two fMRI Experiments. *NeuroImage, 21,* 1320-1336.

Benson, D.F. & Ardila, A. (1996). *Aphasia. A clinical perspective.* New York: Oxford University Press.

Berndt, R. S. & Caramazza, A. (1980). A Redefinition of the Syndrome of Broca's Aphasia: Implications for a Neuropsychological Model of Language. *Applied Psycholinguistics 1*, 225-278.

Berndt, R.S. & Caramazza, A. (1999). How ''Regular'' Is Sentence Comprehension in Broca's Aphasia? It Depends on How You Select the Patients. *Brain and Language, 67*, 242–247

Berndt, R.S., Mitchum, C.C. & Haendiges, M.A. (1996). Comprehension of Reversible Sentences in "Agrammatism": A meta-analysis. *Cognition, 58,* 289-308.

Binkofski, F. & Buccino, G. (2004). Motor functions of the Broca's region. *Brain and Language, 89,* 362-369.

Binkofski, F., Amunts, K., Stephen, K.M., Posse, S., Schormann, T., Freund, H.J., Zilles, K. & Seitz, R.J. (2000). Broca's Region Subserves Imagery of Motion: A Combined Cytoarchitectonic and fMRI Study. *Human Brain Mapping, 11,* 273-285.

Blake, B.J. (1994). *Case.* Cambridge: Cambridge University Press.

Bonilha, L. & Fridriksson, J. (2009). Subcortical damage and white matter disconnection associated with non-fluent speech. *Brain, 132,* 1-2.

Bošković, Ž. (1997). Superiority Effects with Multiple Wh-Fronting in Serbo-Croatian. *Lingua, 102*, 1-20.

Brabec, I., Hraste, M. & Živković, S. (1958). *Gramatika hrvatskoga ili srpskoga jezika.* Zagreb: Školska knjiga.

Broca P. (1861/2001). Remarks on the Seat of the Faculty of Articulate Language, Followed by an Observation of Aphemia. In: Bechtel R, Stffleabeam S,

Mundale J, Manic, P. (Eds.), *Philosophy and the Neurosciences: A Reader*. (87-99). Blackwell Publishers, Oxford.

Brown, K. & Miller, J. (1991). *Syntax: A Linguistic Introduction to Sentence Structure*. London: Harper Collins.

Browne, W. (1986). *Relative Clauses in Serbo-Croatian in Comparison with English*. Zagreb: Institute of Linguistics, University of Zagreb.

Caplan, D. (1995). *Neurolinguistics and linguistic aphasiology. An introduction.* Cambridge: Cambridge University Press.

—. (2001). Measurement of Chance Performance in Aphasia, with Specific Reference to the Comprehension of Semantically Reversible Passive Sentences: A Note on Issues Raised by Caramazza, Capitani, Rey, and Berndt (2001) and Drai, Grodzinsky, and Zurif (2001). *Brain and Language, 76*, 193-201.

—. (2002). The Neural Basis of Syntactic Processing: A Critical Look. In: Hillis, A. (Ed.), *Handbook of Adult Language Disorders*. London: Taylor & Francis.

Caplan, D., Alpert, N., Waters, G. & Olivieri, A. (2000). Activation of Broca's area by syntactic processing under conditions of concurrent articulation. *Human Brain Mapping, 9,* 65-71.

Caplan, D. & Futter, C. (1986). Assignment of Thematic Roles to Nouns in Sentence Comprehension by an Agrammatic Patient. *Brain and Language, 27*, 117-134.

Caplan, D. & Hildebrandt, N. (1988). *Disorders of Syntactic Comprehension.* Cambridge, MA: MIT Press.

Caplan, D., Vijayan, S., Kuperberg, G, West, C., Waters, G., Greve, D. & Dale, A.M. (2001). Vascular Responses to Syntactic Processing: Event Related fMRI Study of Relative Clauses. *Human Brain Mapping, 15,* 26-38.

Caplan, D. & Waters, G. (1995). Aphasic Disorders of Syntactic Comprehension and Working Memory Capacity. *Cognitive Neuropsychology, 12* (6), 637-649.

Caplan, D. & Waters, G.S. (1996). Syntactic Processing in Sentence Comprehension Under Dual-task Conditions in Aphasic Patients. *Language and Cognitive Processes, 11*(5), 525-551.

Caplan, D. & Waters, G. 1999. Verbal Working Memory and Sentence comprehension. *Behavioural and Brain Sciences, 22*, 77-126.

Caplan, D. & Waters, G. (2002). Working Memory and Connectionist Models of Parsing: Reply to MacDonald and Christiansen (2002). *Psychological Review, 109 (1)*, 66-74.

Caramazza, A. & Zurif, E. (1976). Dissociation of Algorithmic and heuristic Processes in Language Comprehension: Evidence from Aphasia. *Brain and Language, 3*, 572-582.

Caramazza, A. & Miceli, G. (1991). Selective Impairment of Thematic Role Assignment in Sentence Processing. *Brain and Language, 41*, 402-436.

Caramazza, A., Capitani, E., Rey, A. Berndt, R.S. (2001). Agrammatic Broca's Aphasia Is Not Associated with a Single Pattern of Comprehension Performance. *Brain and Language, 76*, 158-184.

Chatterjee, A. (2005). A Madness to the Methods in Cognitive Neuroscience? *Journal of Cognitive Neuroscience, 17,* 847-849.

Cheng, L. L-S. (1997). *On the Typology of Wh-Questions*. New York: Garland Publishing, Inc.

Chein, J.M., Ravizza, S.M. & Fiez, J.A. (2003). Using neuroimaging to Evaluate Models of Working Memory and Their Implications for Language Processing. *Journal of Neurolinguistics, 16,* 315-339.

Chomsky, N. (1957). *Syntactic Structures*. Janua Linguarum IV. The Hague: Mouton.

—. (1965). *Aspects of the Theory of Syntax*. Cambridge, MA: MIT Press.

—. (1975). *Reflections on Language*. New York: Pantheon Books.

—. (1981). *Lectures on Government and Binding*. Dordrecht: Foris Publication.

—. (1995). *The Minimalist Program*. Cambridge, MA: The MIT Press.

Cinque, C. (1990). *Types of A' dependencies*. Cambridge, MA: MIT Press.

Clifton, C.; and Frazier, L. (1989). Comprehending sentences with long-distance dependencies. In: Carlson, G.N. & Tanenhaus, M.K *Linguistic Structure in Language Processing* (273-317.). Dordrecht: Kluwer.

Coltheart, M. (2001). Assumptions and methods in cognitive neuropsychology. In Rapp, B. (Ed.) *Handbook of Cognitive Neuropsychology*. New York: Psychology Press.

Comrie, B. (1984). Form and Function in Explaining Language Universals. In: Butterworth, B., Comrie, B. & Dahl, Ö. (Eds.), *Explanations for Language Universals* (87-103). Berlin: Mouton.

Crain, S., Ni, W. & Shankweiler, D. (2001). Grammatism. *Brain and Language, 77*, 294-304.

Crosson, B., Rao, S.M., Woodley, S.J., Rosen, A.C., Bobholz, J.A., Mayer, A., Cunningham, J.M., Hammeke, T.A., Fuller, S.A., Binder, J.R., Cox, R.W. & Stein, E. (1999). Mapping of Semantic, Phonological, and Orthographic Verbal Working Memory in Normal Adults with Functional Magnetic Resonance Imaging. *Neuropsychology, 13*(2), 171-187.

Crystal, D. (1985). *Enciklopedijski rečnik moderne lingvistike. [A Dictionary of Linguistics and Phonetics]* Beograd: Nolit.

Damasio, H. (1991). Neuroanatomical Correlates of the Aphasias. In: Sarno, M.T. (Ed.), *Acquired Aphasia* (pp. 45-71), New York: Academic Press.

Daneman, M. & Carpenter, P. (1980). Individual Differences in Working Memory and Reading. *Journal of Verbal Learning and Verbal Behavior, 19*, 450-466.

Darley, F.L. (1982). *Aphasia*. Philadelphia: W.B. Saunders Company.

Decety, J., Perani, D., Jeannerod, M., Bettinardi, V., Tadardy, B., Woods, R., Mazziotta, J.C. & Fazio, F. (1994). Mapping motor representations with positron emission tomography. *Nature, 371,* 600–602.

Decety, J. & Grèzes, J. (2006). The power of simulation: Imaging one's own and other's behavior. *Brain Research, 1079,* 4-14.

De Rijk, R. (1972). Relative Clauses in Basque: A Guide Tour. *The Chicago Which Hunt:Papers from the Relative Clause Festival.* Chicago Linguistic Society.

De Vincenzi, M. (1996). Syntactic Analysis in Sentence Comprehension: Effects of Dependency Types and Grammatical Constraints. *Journal of Psycholinguistic Research, 25(1),* 117-133.

Drai, D. & Grodzinsky, Y. (1999). Comprehension Regularity in Broca's Aphasia? There's More of It Than You Ever Imagined. *Brain and Language, 70*, 139-143.

Drai, D., Grodzinsky, Y. & Zurif, E. (2001). Broca's Aphasia Is Associated with a Single Pattern of Comprehension Performance: A Reply. *Brain and Language, 76*, 185-192.

Dronkers, N.F., Pinker, S. & Damasio, A. (2000). Language and the Aphasia. In: Kandel, E.R., Schwartz, J.H & Jessell, T.M. (Eds.), *Principles of Neuronal Science* (1169-1187). New York: McGraw-Hill.

Dronkers NF, Plaisant O, Iba-Zizen MT, Cabanis EA. (2007). Paul Broca's historic cases: high resolution MR imaging of the brains of Leborgne and Lelong. *Brain, 130,* 1432-1441.

Dronkers, N.F., Wilkins, D.P., Van Valin, R.D. Jr., Redfern, B.B. & Jaeger, J.J. (1994). A Reconsideration of the Brain Areas Involved in the Disruption of Morphosyntactic Comprehension. *Brain and Language, 47(3),* 461-463.

Druks, J. & Marshall, J.C. (1995). When Passives are Easier than Actives: Two Case Studies of Aphasic Comprehension. *Cognition, 55*, 311-331.

Ehrenkranz, J. & Hirschland, E. C. (1972). Latin Relative Clauses. *The Chicago Which Hunt:Papers from the Relative Clause Festival.* Chicago Linguistic Society.

Embick, D., Marantz, A., Miyashita, Y., O'Neil, W. & Sakai, K.L. (2000). A Syntactic Specialization for Broca's Area. *Proceedings of the National Academy of Sciences of the United States of America,* 97(11), 6150-6154.

Fadiga, L. & Craighero, L. (2006). Hand actions and speech representation in Broca's area.*Cortex, 42,* 486–490.

Fedorenko, E. & Kanwisher, N. (2009). Neuroimaging of Language: Why Hasn't a Clearer Picture Emerged? *Language and Linguistics Compass, 3(4),* 839-865.

Fedorenko, E. Patel, A., Cassanto, D., Winawer, J., & Gibson, E. (2009). Structural integration in language and music: Evidence for a shared system. *Memory and Cognition, 37,* 1–9.

Felser, C., Clahsen, H. & Münte, T.F. (2003). Storage and Integration in the Processing of Filler-Gap Dependencies: An ERP Study of Topicalization and WH-Movement in German. *Brain and Language, 87,* 345-354.

Ferro, J.M. & Madureira, S. (2002). Recovery from cognitive and behavioral deficits. In. Boguslavsky, J. (Ed.), *Long-term effects of stroke* (pp. 140-169). New York: Marcel Dekker, Inc.

Fiebach, C.J., Schlesewsky, M. & Friederici, A.D. (2001). Syntactic Working Memory and the Establishment of Filler-Gap Dependencies: Insights from ERPs and fMRI. *Journal of Psycholinguistic Research, 30,* 321-338.

Fiebach, C.J., Schlesewsky, M., Friederici, A. (2002). Separating Syntactic memory Costs and Integration Costs during Parsing: the Processing of German Wh-questions. *Journal of Memory and Language, 47*, 250-272.

Fiebach, C.J., Schlesewsky, M., Lohmann, G., von Cramon, D.Y & Friederici, A.D. (2004). Revisiting the Role of Broca's Area in Sentence Processing: Syntactic Integration versus Syntactic Working Memory. *Human Brain Mapping, 24,* 79-91.

Fink, G.R., Manjaly, Z.M., Stephen, K.E., Gurd, J.M., Zilles, K., Amunts, K. & Marshall, J.C. (2006). A Role for Broca's Are Beyond Language Processing: Evidence from Neuropsychology and fMRI. In: Amunts, K. & Grodzinsky, Y. (Eds.), *Broca's Region.* Oxford: Oxford University Press.

Fodor, J. A. (1983). *The Modularity of Mind.* Cambridge, MA: The MIT Press.

Frazier, L.& Clifton, C. (1989). Successive cyclicity in the grammar and the parser. *Language and Cognitive Processes, 4.* 93-126.

Frazier, L. & Clifton, C. (2002). Processing "D-linked" phrases. *Journal of Psycholinguistic Research, 31(6),* 633-659.

Frazier, L. & Fodor, J.D. (1978) The sausage machine: A new two-stage parsing model. *Cognition, 6,* 291-325.

Frazier, L. & Friederici, A. (1991). On Deriving the Properties of Agrammatic Comprehension. *Brain and Language, 40,* 51-66.

Frazier, L. & McNamara, P. (1995). Favour Referential Representations. *Brain and Language, 49,* 224-240.

Friederici, A.D. (1998). The Neurobiology of Language Comprehension. In: Friederici, A.D. (Ed.), *Language Comprehension: A Biological Perspective* (pp. 263-301), Berlin: Springer.

Friederici, A.D. & Gorrell, P. (1998). Structural prominence and agrammatic theta-role assignment: A reconsideration of linear strategies. *Brain and Language, 65(2),* 253–275.

Friederici A.D., Rüschemeyer S.A., Hahne A. & Fiebach C.J. (2003). The role of left inferior frontal and superior temporal cortex in sentence comprehension: Localizing syntactic and semantic processes. *Cerebral Cortex, 13,* 170-177.

Friedman, V. (1972). The Relative Clauses in Slavic: South-Slavic. *The Chicago Which Hunt:Papers from the Relative Clause Festival.* Chicago Linguistic Society.

Gaulin, C.A. & Campbell, T. (1994). Procedure for Assessing Verbal Working Memory in Normal School-age Children: Some Preliminary Data. *Perceptual and Motor Skills, 79,* 55-64.

Gazannina, M.S., Ivry, R.B. & Mangun, G.R. (1998). *Cognitive Neuroscience - The Biology of Mind.* New York: W.W. Norton & Company.

Gibson, E. (1998). Linguistic Complexity: Locality of Syntactic Dependencies. *Cognition, 68,* 1–76.

Gibson, E. & Hickok, G. (1993). Sentence Processing with Empty Categories. *Language and Cognitive Processes, 8(2),* 147-161.

Gleason, J.B., Goodglass, H., Green, E., Ackerman, N. & Hyde, M.R. (1975). The retrieval of syntax in Broca's aphasia. *Brain and Language, 2,* 451-457.

Golab, Z. (1972). The Relative Clauses in Slavic: Common Slavic and North Slavic. *The Chicago Which Hunt:Papers from the Relative Clause Festival.* Chicago Linguistic Society.

Gorrell, P. (1993). Evaluating the Direct Association Hypothesis. A Reply to Pickering and Barry (1991). *Language and Cognitive Processes, 8(2),* 129-146.

Goodglass, H. (1993). *Understanding Aphasia.* San Diego: Academic Press, Inc.

Goodglass, H. & Kaplan, E. (1983). *The Assessment of Aphasia and Related Disorders. Philadelphia*: Lea & Febiger.

Greenlee, J.D.W., Oya, H., Kawasaki, H., Volkov, I.O., Severson, A.M., Howard, M.A. & Brugge, J.F. (2007). Functional Connections within the Human Inferior Frontal Gyrus. *The Journal of Comparative Neurology, 503,* 550-559.

Greewe, T., Bornkessel, I., Zysset, S., Wiese, R., von Cramon, Y.D., Schlesewsky, M. (2005). The Emergence of the Unmarked: A New Perspective on the Language-Specific Function of Broca's Area, *Human Brain Mapping, 26*, 178–190.

Grodzinsky, Y. (1984). The syntactic characterization of agrammatism. *Cognition, 16,* 99-120.

—. (1986). Language Deficits and the Theory of Syntax. *Brain and Language, 27,* 135-159.

—. (1990). *Theoretical Perspectives on Language Deficits.* Philadelphia, PA: Lea & Febiger.

—. (1993). Introduction. *Brain and Language, 45*, 299-305.

—. (1995). A Restrictive Theory of Trace Deletion in Agrammatism. *Brain and Language, 50*, 27-51.

—. (2000a). Overarching Agrammatism. In: Grodzinsky, Y., Shapiro, L. & Swinney, D. (Eds.), *Language and the Brain* (pp. 73-86). San Diego: Academic Press.

—. (2000b). The Neurology of Syntax: Language Use without Broca's Area. *Behavioral and Brain Sciences, 23* (1), 1-21.

—. (2010). The Picture of the Linguistic Brain: How Sharp Can It Be? Reply to Fedorenko & Kanwisher. *Language and Linguistics Compass, 4/8*, 605-622.

Grodzinsky, Y., Wexler, K., Chien, Y.C., Marakovitz, S. & Solomon, J. (1993). The Breakdown of Binding Relations, *Brain and Language, 45*, 396-422.

Grodzinsky, Y., Pinango, M. M., Zurif, E., Drai, D. (1999). The Critical Role of Group Studies in Neuropsychology: Comprehension Regularities in Broca's Aphasia. *Brain and Language, 67*, 134-147.

Hagoort, P. 2005. Broca's Complex as the Unification Space for Language In: Cutler A (ed). *Twenty-First Century Psycholinguistics. Four Cornerstones* (pp. 157-172). Mahwah, NJ: Lawrence Erlbaum Associates.

Haarman, H.J., Just, M.A., & Carpenter, P.A. 1997. Aphasic Sentence Comprehension as a Resource Deficit: A Computational Approach. *Brain and Language, 59*, 76-120.

Haarmann, H.J. & Kolk, H. (1991). Syntactic priming in Broca's aphasics: evidence for slow activation. *Aphasiology, 5*, 247-263.

Haegemen, L. (1991). *Introduction to Government & Binding Theory*. Basil Blackwell.

Hagiwara, H. (1993). The breakdown of Japanese passives and theta-role assignment principle by Broca's aphasics. *Brain and Language, 45,* 318–339.

—. (1995). The breakdown of functional categories and the economy of derivation. *Brain and Language, 50(1)*, 92-116.

Haines, D.E. (2008). *Neuroanatomy. An Atlas of Structures, Sections, and Systems.* Philadelphia: Wolters Kluwer. (Seventh edition).

Hawkins, J.A. (1999). Processing Complexity and Filler-Gap Dependencies across Grammars. *Language, 75(2),* 244-285.

Hauser, R. R. (1983). The Syntax and Semantics of English Mood. *Questions and Answers*. Dordrecht: D. Reidel Publishing Company.

Heeschen, C. & Kolk, H. (1988). Agrammatism and Paragrammatism. *Aphasiology, 2,* 299-302.

Hickok, G., Zurif, E., Canseco-Gonzales, E. (1993). Structural Description of Agrammatic Comprehension. *Brain and Language, 45*, 371-395.

Hickok, G. & Avrutin, S. (1993). Representation, Referentiality, and Processing in Agrammatic Comprehension: Two Case Studies. *Brain and Language, 50*, 10-26.

Hickok, G. & Avrutin, S. (1996). Comprehension of Wh-Questions in Two Broca's Aphasics. *Brain and Language, 52*, 314-327.

Hickok, G. & Poeppel, D. (2000). Towards a Functional Anatomy of Speech Perception. *Trends in Cognitive Sciences, 4,* 131-138.

Hickok, G. & Poeppel, D. (2004). Dorsal and ventral streams: a framework for understanding aspects of the functional anatomy of language. *Cognition, 92,* 67-99.

Hickok, G. & Poeppel, D. (2007).The cortical organization of speech processing. *Nature Reviews Neuroscience, 8,* 393-402.

Hillis, A. (2007). Aphasia: Progress in the last quarter of a century. *Neurology, 69,* 200-213.

Inglis, A.L. (1999). The Complexity of 'Asyntactic' Comprehension: Investigations of an Unusual Dissociation Between Passives and Object Relatives. *Journal of Neurolinguistics, 12*, 41-77.

Jackendoff, R. (1997). *The Architecture of the Language Faculty*. Cambridge, MA: The MIT Press.

—. (2000). Fodorian Modularity and Representational Modularity. In: Grodzinsky, Y., Shapiro, L. & Swinney, D. (Eds.), *Language and the Brain. Representation and Processing* (pp. 4-30). San Diego: Academic Press.

—. (2002). *Foundations of Language. Brain, Meaning, Grammar, Evolution.* Oxford: Oxford University Press.

Jonides, J. & Smith, E.E. (1997). The Architecture of Working Memory. In: Rugg, M.D. (Ed.), *Cognitive Neuroscience*. Cambridge, MA: The MIT Press.

Just, M. & Carpenter, P. (1992). A Capacity Theory of Comprehension: Individual Differences in Working Memory. *Psychological Review, 99*, 122-149.

Just, M. A. & Varma, S. (2002). A Hybrid Architecture for Working Memory: Reply to MacDonald and Christiansen (2002). *Psychological Review, 109*, 55-65.

Just, M.A., Carpenter, P.A., Keller, T.A., Eddy, W.F. & Thulborn, K.R. (1996). Brain Activation Modulated by Sentence Comprehension. *Science, 274 (5284)*, 114-116.

Kaan, E. & Stowe, L.A. (2002). Storage and computation in sentence processing: A neurimaging perspective. In: Noteboom, S,G., Weerman, F. & Wijnen, F. (Eds.), *Storage and Computation in the Language Faculty* (pp. 257-298). Dordrecht: Kluwer.

Kaan, E. & Swaab, T.Y. (2002). The brain circuitry of syntactic comprehension. *TRENDS in Cognitive Sciences, 6(8),* 350–356.

Kang, A.M., Constable, R.T., Gore, J.C. & Avrutin, S. (1999). An Event-Related fMRI Study of Implicit Phrase-Level Syntactic and Semantic Processing. *NeuroImage, 10*, 555-561.

Karbe, H, Thiel, A., Weber-Luxenburger, G., Herholz, K., Kessler, J. & Heiss, W.D. (1998). Brain Plasticity in Poststroke Aphasia: What is the Contribution of the Right Hemisphere? *Brain and Language, 64*, 215–30.

Karttunen, L. (1978). Syntax and Semantics of Questions. *Questions*. Dordrecht: D. Reidel Publishing Company.

Katz, L., Rexer, K. & Peter, M. (1995). Case Morphology and Thematic Rol in Word Recognition. In: Feldman, L.B. (Ed.), *Morphological Aspects of Language Processing* (pp. 79-107). Hillsdale, NJ: Lawrence Erlbaum Associates, Publishers.

Kean, M-L. (1995). The Elusive Character of Agrammatism. *Brain and Language, 50*, 369-384.

Keenan, E.L. & Comrie, B. (1977). Noun Phrase Accessibility and Universal Grammar. *Linguistic Inquiry, 8(1),* 63-100.

Keller, T.A., Carpenter, P.A. & Just. M.A. (2001). The Neural Bases of Sentence Comprehension: a fMRI Examination of Syntactic and lexical Processing. *Cerebral Crotex, 11* (3), 223-237.

Kempe, V. & MacWhinney, B. (1999). Processing of Morphological and Semantic Cues in Russian and German. *Language and Cognitive Processes, 14(2),* 129-171.

Kempen, G. (1998). Sentence parsing. In: Friederici, A.D. (Ed.), *Language Comprehension: A Biological Perspective* (pp. 211-227), Berlin: Springer.

Kennedy, M. M. & Small, J. A. (2002). *On the Domain Specificity of the Resources for Sentence Processing*. Ms. School of Audiology and Speech Sciences, University of British Columbia.

Kertesz, A. & McCabe, P. (1975). Intelligence and aphasia: Performance of aphasics on Raven's Coloured Progressive Matrices (RCPM). *Brain and Language, 2,* 387-395.

King, J.W. & Kutas, M. (1995) Who Did What and When? Using Word- and Clause-level ERPs to Monitor Working Memory Usage in Reading. *Journal of Cognitive Neuroscience, 7(3),* 376-395.

Kljajevic, V. (2011a). Language Reorganization after Stroke: Insights from fMRI. In: Rakesh R. Sharma (Ed.), *Functional Magnetic Resonance Imaging,* Book 2, Rijeka: InTech.

—. (2011b). Broca's Area: Four Misconceptions. *Current Topics in Neurology, Psychiatry and Related Disciplines, 19(1), 20-30.*

Kljajevic, V. & Bastiaanse, R. (2011). Time reference in fluent aphasia: Evidence from Serbian. In: Vatakis, A., Cumminis, F., Esposito, A., Papadelis, G. & Giagkou, M. (Eds.) *Multidisciplinary Aspects of Time and Time Perception* (pp. 258-274). Berlin: Springer.

Kljajevic, V. & Fratini, V. (2011). *Comprehension of wh-dependencies in elderly: Evidence from Spanish.* Unpublished study. San Sebastian: Insituto Gerontológico Matia.

Kljajevic, V.& Murasugi, K. (2010). The role of morphology in the comprehension of wh-dependencies in Croatian aphasic speakers. *Aphasiology, 24,* 1354-1376.
Kluender, R. & Kutas. M. (1993) Subjacency as a Processing Phenomena. *Language and Cognitive Processes, 8,* 573-633.
Kolk, H. (1995). A Time-Based Approach to Agrammatic Production. *Brain and Language, 50*, 282-303.
Kolk, H. & Heeschen, C. (1990). Adaptation symptoms and impairment symptoms in Broca's aphasia. *Aphasiology, 4,* 221-231.
Kordić, S. (1995). *Relativna rečenica*. Zagreb: Matica Hrvatska.
Kotz, S.A. & Friederici, A.D. (2003). Electrophysiology of Normal and Pathological Language Processing. *Journal of Neurolinguistics, 16* (1), 43-58.
Kutas, M., Federmeier, K.D., Coulson, S., King, J.W. & Münte, T.F. (2000). Language. In: Cacioppo, J.T, Tassinary, L.G. & Berntson, G. *Handbook of Psychophysiology* (pp. 576-600). Cambridge: Cambridge University Press.
Lasnik, H. & Uriagereka, J. (1988). *A Course in GB Syntax*. Cambridge, MA: The MIT Press.
Lewis, R. L. (1999). Accounting for the Fine Structure of Syntactic Working Memory: Similarity-Based Interface as a Unifying Principle. *Behavioral and Brain Sciences, 22*, 105-106.
Linebarger, M.C., Schwartz, M.F. & Saffran, E.M. (1983). Sensitivity to Grammatical Structure in so-called Agrammatic Aphasics. *Cognition, 13*, 361-392.
Lindenberg, R., Fangerau, H., Seitz, R.J. (2007). "Broca's area" as a collective term? *Brain and Language, 102,* 22-29.
Lukatela, K. (1989). *Sentence Processing in Fluent and Non-Fluent Aphasia.* Dissertation. The University of Connecticut.
Lukatela, K., Crain, S. & Shankweiler, D. (1988). Sensitivity to Inflectional Morphology in Agrammatism: Investigation of a Highly Inflected Language. *Brain and Language, 33*, 1-15.
Lukatela, K., Shankweiler, D. & Crain, S. (1995). Syntactic Processing in Agrammatic Aphasia by Speakers of a Slavic Language. *Brain and Language, 49,* 50-76.
MacWhinney, B. (1987). The Competition Model. In: MacWhinney, B. (Ed.), *Mechanisms of Language Acquisition* (pp. 249-308). Hillsdale, NJ: Lawrence Erlbaum Associates, Publishers.
Maess, B., Koelsch, S., Gunter, T. & Friederici, A. (2001). Musical syntax is processed in Broca's area: an MEG study. *Nature Neuroscience, 4,* 540-545.
Marchand, Y., D'Arcy, R.C.N. & Connoly, J.F. (2002). Linking Neurophysiological and Neuropsychological Measures for Aphasia Assessment. *Clinical Neurophysiology, 113(11),* 1715-1722.
Martin, R. (1995). Working Memory Doesn't Work: A Critique of Miyake et al.'s Capacity Theory of Aphasic Comprehension Deficits. *Cognitive Neuropsychology, 12* (6), 623-636.
Martin, R.C. & Miller, M.D. (2002). Sentence comprehension deficits: Independence and interaction of syntax, semantics, and working memory. In:

Hillis, A. (Ed.), *Handbook of Adult Language Disorders: Integrating Cognitive Neuropsychology, Neurology, and Rehabilitation*. New York: Psychology Press.

Martin, R.C. & Romani, C. (1994). Verbal Working Memory and Sentence Comprehension: A Multiple-Components View. *Neuropsychology, 8(4),* 506-523.

Mauner, G., Fromkin, V.A. & Cornell, T.L. (1993). Comprehension of acceptability judgment in agrammatism: Disruption in the syntax of referential dependency. *Brain and Language, 45,* 340-370.

Mauner, G. (1995). Examining the Empirical and Linguistic Bases of Current Theories of Agrammatism. *Brain and Language*, *50*, 339-368.

McCawley, J.D. (1972). Japanese Relative Clauses. *The Chicago Which Hunt:Papers from the Relative Clause Festival.* Chicago Linguistic Society.

Milekic, S. (1993). *Distance and Position Effects in Sentence Processing by Agrammatic Aphasics*. Dissertation. The University of Connecticut.

Miyake, A., Carpenter, P., & Just, M.A. (1994). A Capacity Approach to Syntactic Comprehension Disorders: Making Normal Adults Perform like Aphasic Patients. *Cognitive Neuropsychology, 11*(6), 671-717.

Miyake, A., Carpenter, P., & Just, M.A. (1995). Reduced Resources and Specific Impairments in Normal and Aphasic Sentence Comprehension. Cognitive *Neuropsychology, 12* (6), 651-679.

Mohr, J.P. (1976). Broca's area and Broca's aphasia. In: Whitaker H. & Whitaker, HA (Eds.), *Studies in Neurolinguistics.* Academic Press (201-235), New York.

Müller, H.M., King, J.W. & Kutas, M. (1997). Event-related potentials elicited by spoken relative clauses. *Cognitive Brain Research, 5,* 193-203.

Münte, T.F. & Heinze, H.-J. (1994). ERP Negativities During Syntactic Processing of Written Words. In: Heinze, H.-J, Münte, T.F. & Mangun, G.R. (Eds.), *Cognitive Electrophysiology* (pp. 211-38). Boston: Birkhäuser.

Murray, L. (1999). Attention and Aphasia: Theory, Research and Clinical Implications. *Aphasiology, 13(2),* 91-111.

Nadau, S.E. & Crosson, B. (1997). Subcortical Aphasia. *Brain and Language, 58,* 355-402.

Naeser, M.A., Martin, P., Nicholas, M., Baker, E.H., Seekins, H., Helm-Estabrooks, N. et al. (2005). Improved naming after TMS treatments in a chronic, global aphasia patient—case report. *Neurocase, 11(3),* 182–193

Nagai, C., Inui, T. & Iwata, M. (2010). Role of Broca's Subregions in Syntactic Processing: A Comparative Study of Japanese Patients with Lesions in the Pars Triangularis and Opercularis. *European Neurology, 63,* 79-86.

Neuhaus, E., & Penke, M. (2008). Production and comprehension of wh-questions in German Broca's aphasia. *Journal of Neurolinguistics, 21*, 150–176.

Nikolić, S. (1983). *Staroslovenski jezik.* Beograd: Naučna knjiga.

Noordman, L.G.M. & Vonk, W. (1999) Discourse Comprehension In: Friederici, A.D. (Ed.), *Language Comprehension: A Biological Perspective* (pp. 229-262). Berlin: Springer.

Novick, J.M., Trueswell, J.C., Thompson-Schill, S.L. (2005). Cognitive control and parsing: Reexamining the role of Broca's area in sentence comprehension. *Cognitive Affective, & Behavioral Neuroscience, 5(3),* 263-281.

Novick, J.M., Trueswell, J.C., Thompson-Schill, S.L. (2010). Broca's Area and Language Processing: Evidence for the Cognitive Control Connection, *Language and Linguistics Compass, 4(10)*, 906-924.

Ojemann, G.A. (1991). Cortical Organization of Language. *The Journal of Neuroscience, 11(8),* 2281-2287.

Optiz B. & Friederici A.D..(2007). Neural Basis of Processing Sequential and Hierarchical Syntactic Structures. *Human Brain Mapping, 28*, 585-592.

Paradis, M. (2001). The need for awareness of aphasia symptoms in different languages. *Journal of Neurolinguistics, 14,* 85–91.

Pascual-Leone, A., Amedi, A., Fregni, F. &. Merabet, L.B. (2005). The Plastic Human Brain Cortex. *Annual Review of Neuroscience, 28,* 377–401

Patel, A. (2003). Language, music, syntax and the brain. *Nature Neuroscience,* 7, 674–681.

Patel, A. (2008). *Music, Language, and the Brain.* Oxford: Oxford University Press.

Pesetsky, D. (1987). *Wh*-in situ. Movement and Unselective Binding. Reuland, E. & ter Meulen, A. (Eds.), *The Representations of (In)definiteness* (pp. 98-129). Cambridge, Mass: MIT Press.

Peterson, K.M., Forkstam, C. & Ingvar, M. (2004). Artificial syntactic violations activate Broca's area. *Cognitive Science, 28,* 383-407.

Petrides, M., Alivisatos, B., Meyer, E. & Evans, A.C., (1993). Functional Activation of the Human Frontal Cotrex during the Performance of Verbal Working Memory Tasks. *Proceedings of the National Academy of Science USA, 90*, 878-882.

Pickering, M. (1993). Direct Association and Sentence Processing: A Reply to Gorrell and to Gibson and Hickok. *Language and Cognitive Processes, 8(2),* 163-196.

Pickering, M. & Barry, G. (1991). Sentence Processing without Empty Categories. *Language and Cognitive Processes, 6,* 229-259.

Piñango, M.P. (2000a). Canonicity in Broca's Sentence Comprehension: The Case of Psychological Verbs. In: Grodzinsky, Y., Shapiro, L. & Swinney, D. *Language and the Brain* (pp. 327-350), San Diego: Academic Press.

—. (2000b). Syntactic Displacement in Broca's Agrammatic Aphasia.In: Bastiaanse, R. & Grodzinsky, Y. (Eds.). *Grammatical Disorders in Aphasia. A Neurolinguistic Perspective* (75-87). London: Whur Publishers.

Platzack, C. (2000). Multiple Interfaces. In: Van der Zee & Nikanne, U. (Eds.). *Cognitive Interfaces. Constraints on Linking Cognitive Information* (pp. 21-54). Oxford: Oxford University Press.

Poeppel, D. & Embick, D. (2005). Defining the relation between linguistics and neuroscience. In: Cutler, A. (Ed.), Twenty-First Century Psycholinguistics. Four Cornerstones (pp. 103-120). Mahwah, NJ.: Lawrence Erlbaum Associates.

Poldrack, R.A., Temple, E., Protopapas, A., Nagarajan, S., Tallal, P., Merzenich, M., & Gabrieli, J.D. (2001). Relations between the neural basis of dynamic auditory processing and phonological processing: Evidence from fMRI. *Journal of Cognitive Neuroscience, 13(5)*, 687-697.

Poldrack, R.A., Wagner, A.D., Prull, M.W., Desmond, J.E., Glover, H.G. & Gabrieli, J.D.E. (1999). Functional Specialization for Semantic and Phonological Processing in the Left Inferior Premotor Cortex. *NeuroImage, 10,* 15-35.

Price, C.J. (1998). The Functional Anatomy of Word Comprehension and Production. *Trends in Cognitive Science, 2,* 281-288

—. (2010). The anatomy of language: a review of 100 fMRI studies *Annals of the New York Academy of Sciences, 1191,* 62-88.

Prather, P., Shapiro, L., Zurif, E. & Swinney, D. (1991). Real-Time Examinations of Lexical Processing in Aphasics. *Journal of Psycholinguistic Research, 20(3),* 271-282.

Progovac, Lj. (1996). Clitics in Serbian/Croatian: Comp as the Second Position. In: Halpern, A.L. & Zwicky, A.M. (Eds.). *Approaching Second: Second Position Clitics and Related Phenomena* (pp. 411-428). Stanford, CA: CSLI Publications.

Pulvermüller, F. (2010). Brain-Language Research: Where is the Progress? *Biolinguistics, 4(2-3),* 255-288.

Raven, J. C. (1965). *Coloured progressive matrices.* London: H.K. Lewis & Co.

Raven, J.C., Court, J.H., & Raven, J. (1976). *Manual for Raven's Progressive Matrices and Vocabulary Scales.* London: H. K. Lewis & Co. Ltd.

Reinvang, I. (1985). *Aphasia and brain organization.* New York: Plenum Press.

Rösler, F., Pechmann, T., Streb, J., Röder, B. & Hennighausen, E. (1998) Parsing of Sentences in a Language with Varying Word Order: Word-by-Word Variations of Processing Demands are Revealed by Event Related Potentials. *Journal of Memory and Language, 38,* 150-176.

Rudin, C. (1988). On Multiple Questions and Multiple *Wh* Fronting. *Natural Language and Linguistic Theory, 6*, 445-501.

Saffran, E. (2000). The Organization of Semantic Memory: In Support of a Distributed Model. *Brain and Language, 71*, 204-212.

Sakai, K.L., Noguchi, Y., Takeuchi, T. & Watanabe, E. (2002). Selective Priming of Syntactic Processing by Event-Related Transcranial Magnetic Stimulation of Broca's Area. *Neuron, 35,* 1177-1182.

Salis, C. & Edwards, S. (2008). Comprehension of *wh*-questions and declarative sentences in agrammatic aphasia: The set partition hypothesis. *Journal of Neurolinguistics, 21,* 375–399.

Saur, D., Lange, R., Baumgaertner, A., Schraknepper, V., Willmes, K., et al. (2006). Dynamics of language reorganization after stroke. *Brain, 129*, 1371-1384.

Schacter, D. & Tulving, E. (1994) *Memory Systems.* Cambridge, MA: MIT Press.

Silva-Pereyra, J., Conboy, B. T., Klarman, L. & Kuhl, P. K. (2007). Grammatical Processing without Semantics? An Event-Related Brain Potential Study of Preeschoolers using Jabberwocky Sentences. *Journal of Cognitive Neuroscience, 19,* 1050-1065.

Slack, J.M. (2000). Temporal Bounds on Interfaces. In: Van der Zee, E. & Nikanne, U. *Cognitive Interfaces. Constraints on Linking Cognitive Information* (pp. 215-234). Oxford: Oxford University Press.

Smith, S.D. & Mimica, I. (1984). Agrammatism in a Case-Inflected Language: Comprehension of Agent-Object Relations. *Brain and Language, 21*, 274-290.

Spreen, O. & Risser, A.H. (2003). *Assesment of Aphasia.* Oxford: Oxford University Press.

Stevanović, M. (1981). *Savremeni srpskohrvatski jezik.* Beograd: Naučna knjiga.

Stjepanovic, S. (1999). *What Do Second Position Cliticization, Scrambling and Multiple Wh-Fronting Have in Common?* Dissertation. The University of Connecticut.

Stowe, L.A. (1989). Thematic Structures and Sentence Comprehension. In: Carlson, G.N. & Tanenhaus, M.K. (Eds.), *Linguistic Structures in Language Processing* (pp. 319-357). Dordrecht: Kluwer Academic Publishers.

Stowe, L.A., Withaar, R.G., Wijers, A.A., Broere, C.A.J. & Paans, A.M.J. (2002). Encoding and Storage in Working Memory during Sentence Comprehension. In: Merlo, P. & Stevenson, S. (Eds.), *The Lexical Basis of Sentence Processing.* Amsterdam: John Benjamins Publishing Company.

Strelnikov, K. N., Vorobyev, V.A., Chernigovskaya, T.V. & Medvedev, S.V. (2006). Prosodic clues to syntactic processing—a PET and ERP study. *NeuroImage, 29*, 1127-1134.

Stromswold, K., Caplan, D., Alpert, N. & Rauch, S. (1996). Localization of Syntactic Comprehension by Positron Emission Tomography. *Brain and Language, 52*, 452-473.

Swaab, T., Brown, C. & Hagoort, P. (1997). Spoken Sentence Comprehension in Aphasia: Event-related Potential Evidence for a Lexical Integration Deficit. *Journal of Cognitive Neuroscience, 9* (1), 39-66.

Swinney, D. & Zurif, E. (1993). Syntactic Processing in Aphasia. *Brain and Language, 50*, 225-239.

Swinney, D., Zurif, E., Prather, P. & Love, T. (1996). Neurological Distribution of Processing Resources Underlying Language Comprehension. *Journal of Cognitive Neuroscience, 8(2),* 174-184.

Tagashira, Y. (1972). Relative Clauses in Korean. *The Chicago Which Hunt:Papers from the Relative Clause Festival.* Chicago Linguistic Society.

Tait, M.E., Thompson, C.K. & Ballard, K.J. (1995). Subject/Object Asymmetries in Agrammatic Comprehension of Four Types of *Wh*-Questions. Academy of Aphasia Conference.*Brain and Language, 51,* 77-79.

Thomson, A.J. & Martinet, A.V. (1997). *A Practical English Grammar.* Oxford: Oxford University Press.

Thompson, C.K., Tait, M.E., Ballard, K.J. & Fix, S.C. (1999). Agrammatic Aphasic Subjects Comprehension of Subject and Object Extracted *Wh*-Questions. *Brain and Language, 67*, 169-187.

Thompson-Schill SL. (2005). Dissecting the Language Organ: A new Look at the Role of Broca's Area in Language Processing. In: Cutler, A. (Ed.), *Twenty-First Century Psycholinguistics. Four Cornerstones* (pp. 173-190). Mahwah, NJ.: Lawrence Erlbaum Associates.

Tłokiński, W. (1995). Linguistic Competence, Experience and Agrammatism. *Aphasiology.* Vol. 9, No 2, pp. 137-142.

Tonkonogy, J. (1986). *Vascular Aphasia.* Cambridge, MA: MIT Press.

Townsend, D.J. & Bever, T.G. (2001). *Sentence Comprehension: The Integration of Habits and Rules*. Cambridge, MA.:MIT Press

Tranel, D. & Damasio, A.R. (1995). Neurobiological Foundations of Human Memory. *Handbook of Memory Disorders.*

Tulving, E. (1972). Episodic and Semantic Memory. In: Tulving, E. & Donaldson, W. (Eds.), *Organization of Memory* (pp. 381-403). New York: Academic Press.

Turken, A.U. & Dronkers, N.F. (2011). The neural architecture of the language comprehension network: converging evidence from lesion and connectivity analysis. *Frontiers in Systems Neuroscience, 5,* 1-20.

Ueno, M. (2003). *Event-related Brain Potentials in the Processing of Japanese Wh-Questions.* PhD thesis. University of California, San Diego.

Ulatowska, H.K., Sadowska, D. & Kądzielawa, D. (2001). A longitudinal study of agrammatism in Polish : A case study. *Journal of Neurolinguistics, 14*, 321-336.

Uttal, W.R. (2001). *The New Phrenology. The Limits of Localizing Cognitive Processes in the Brain.* Cambridge, MA.: The MIT Press.

Van der Linden, M. & Poncelat, M. (1998). The Role of Working Memory in Language and Communication Disorders. In: Stemmer, B. & Whitaker, H. (Eds.). *Handbook of Neurolinguistics* (pp. 289-300). San Diego: Academic Press.

Van der Meulen, I., Bastiaanse, R. & Rooryck, J. (2005). Wh-questions in agrammatism: a movement deficit? *Stem-, Spraak- en Taalpathologie, 13,* 24-36.

Vignolo, L.A. (1988). The Anatomical and Pathological Basis of Aphasia. In: Rose, C.F., Whurr, R. & Wyke, M.A. (Eds.), *Aphasia* (pp. 227-249). London: Whurr Publishers.

Vos, S.H., Gunter, T.C., Schriefers, H. & Friederici, A.D. (2001). Syntactic Parsing and Working Memory: The Effects of Syntactic Complexity, Reading Span, and Concurrent Load. *Language and Cognitive Processes, 16* (1), 65-103.

Wechsler, D. (1981). *Wechsler Adult Intelligence Scale—Revised.* Cleveland, Ohio: The Psychological Corp.

Whitaker. H.A. (1997) Some Comments on Pre-modern Agrammatism Research. In: Whitaker, H.A. (Ed.) *Agrammatism* (pp. 1-8). San Diego: Singular Press.

Willmes, K. & Poeck, K. (1993). To what extent can aphasic syndromes be localized? *Brain, 116,* 1527-1540.

Wise, R.J.S., Scott, S.K., Blank, C.S., Mummery, C.J., Murphy, K. & Warburton, E. (2001). Separate neural subsystems within 'Wernicke's area'. *Brain, 124,* 83-95.

van der Zee, E. & Nikanne, U. (2000). Introducing Cognitive Interfaces and Constraints on Linking Cognitive Information. In: Van der Zee, E. & Nikanne, U. (Eds.), *Cognitive Interfaces. Constrains on Linking Cognitive Information* (pp. 1-21). Oxford: Oxford University Press.

Zurif, E.B. (1995). Brain Regions of Relevance to Syntactic Processing. Second edition. Gleitman, L. & Liberman, M. (Eds.), *An Invitation to Cognitive Science. Language.* (381-397) Cambridge, MA.: MIT Press.

Zurif, E., Swinney, D., Prather, P., Solomon, J. & Bushell, C. (1993). An On-Line Analysis of Syntactic Processing in Broca's and Wernicke's Aphasia. *Brain and Language, 45*, 448-464.

Zurif, E. & Piñango, M.M. (1999). The Existence of Comprehension Patterns in Broca's Aphasia. *Brain and Language, 70*, 133-138.

INDEX